Juliet Leigh is the author of *The Baby Bible*. She is a mother of two and lives in London.

Also by Juliet Leigh

The Baby Bible

THE BEST BABY BUYS GUIDE

The Essential Handbook for Every New Parent

Juliet Leigh

HEADLINE

Copyright © 1999 Juliet Leigh

The right of Juliet Leigh to be identified as the Author of the Work has been asserted by her in accordance with the Copyright, Designs and Patents Act 1988.

First published in 1999
by HEADLINE BOOK PUBLISHING

10 9 8 7 6 5 4 3 2 1

All rights reserved. No part of this publication may be reproduced, stored in a retrieval system, or transmitted, in any form or by any means without the prior written permission of the publisher, nor be otherwise circulated in any form of binding or cover other than that in which it is published and without a similar condition being imposed on the subsequent purchaser.

ISBN 0 7472 7613 7

Typeset by
Letterpart Limited, Reigate, Surrey

Printed and bound in Great Britain by
Mackays of Chatham PLC, Chatham, Kent

HEADLINE BOOK PUBLISHING
A division of Hodder Headline PLC
338 Euston Road
London NW1 3BH

This book is dedicated with gratitude to the parents, carers and industry professionals who generously gave up their time to help on this project.

Publisher's Note

The views expressed within this book are the author's own, based on her own research and on the views of other organisations. Before buying a particular product, you should obviously check it very carefully. You should also bear in mind that views on which products are appropriate for babies change over time. The publishers and the author do not therefore take responsibility for any injury which may occur as a result of using any of the products recommended within this book.

Contents

Acknowledgements	ix
Preface	1
Introduction	3
Section 1: The Bare Necessities	17
Baby Clothes	19
Baths	29
Bath Products	34
Bottle Feeding	36
Sterilisers	43
Bottle-Feeding Accessories	48
Soothers/Dummies	51
Breastfeeding Bras	53
Breastfeeding Accessories	59
Breast Pumps	62
Changing Units and Mats	65
Cots and Cot Beds	69
Cot Mattresses	75
Baby Bedding	79
Moses Baskets	83
Medicine Cabinet	86
Monitors	89
Nappies	94
Disposable Nappies	95
Reusable Nappies	98
Changing Accessories	101
Car Seats	103
Car Seat Accessories	111
Pushchairs and Buggies	114
Prams	123
Convertibles, Combinations and Travel Systems	125
Double Buggies	132
All-Terrain Buggies	135

Holidays with a Baby	137
Section 2: Optional Extras	**147**
Baby Bouncers	149
Baby Walkers	152
Baby Carriers	153
Baby Chairs	158
Books	162
Videos	169
Multimedia	171
Changing Bags	172
Cycling with a Baby	176
Nursery Furnishings	181
Toys	189
Travel Cots	199
Section 3: Necessities for Older Babies	**203**
Baby Food and Feeding Accessories	205
Bowls, Spoons and Cups	210
Bibs	215
Highchairs	217
Potties and Toilet Training Aids	224
Safety Gadgets	228
Gates and Barriers	237
Shoes	242
Teeth and Dental Care	244
General Baby Goods Suppliers	**248**
Regional Retailers	**252**
Index	**266**
Readers' Report Form	**275**

Acknowledgements

This project turned out to be more of a marathon than anyone expected. I am therefore indebted to Andrew Lownie, who kicked me towards the starting post; Heather Holden-Brown, who bravely put me under starter's orders; and Lindsay Symons who kept up an intelligent commentary throughout. Kelly Davis, Jane Selley and Jayne Booth yanked me down the final furlong to the finish line – what a team – thank you.

Thank you also to Robert Chantry-Price for being unfailingly kind and helpful.

Stephen Parker, thank you, *thank you*, for putting up with me for the duration . . . you are definitely worthy of a Best Baby Buys Gold Star. Tina, I couldn't have done with this without your calm and meticulous assistance. Kate, your help and expert views have been invaluable. Trevor – you did so much to help me, I don't know how to start thanking you either but I'm sure you'll think of a way! Tom and Annabel – my original little guinea pigs have now grown into large monkeys but I am grateful to them and all the children, babies and their carers whose lively commitment to this project made it such fun.

Additional research organised by:
Tina Grant-Brook (senior researcher), Jessica Bondy, Kate Jones in London and the West Country.

Regional research co-ordinators:

Jacqui Bealing, South Coast
Anna Collins, North East
Caroline Culot, East Anglia
Sharon Dale, Yorkshire
Angela Epstein, Manchester
Jane Gallagher, Liverpool

Joan McFadden, Glasgow and the Scottish Highlands
Anna Morrell, Wales
Ruth Walker, Edinburgh and locality
Graham Young, Birmingham

Expert opinions kindly given by:

Robert Chantry-Price, Baby Products Association
Fiona Hockenhull, Area Manager, Teddies Nurseries
Kate Jewitt, Child Accident Prevention Trust
Julia Rowley and the Healthcare team, Boots the Chemist
Samantha Sherratt, Foundation for the Study of Infant Deaths
Gina Siddons, TAMBA
Susan Tanner, A. Dawood & S. Tanner Dental Practice
Rainey Waldorf, ABC Nursery Supplies
Alison Watts, National Childbirth Trust
Marianne Williams

Whilst I am extremely grateful for the invaluable assistance of these experts, I would like to make it clear that the views expressed in this book are my own.

The following also gave of their time and expertise:
Caroline Lucas, Christine McGrigor, Katie Sunley, Sue Newell, Pandora Brady, Mark Jones, Victoria Elton, Nick Green, Howard Burrell, Victoria Squires, Liz Sheinman, Beverley Tilitser, Samantha Paine, Kelly St Cyr, Penny Ainge, Annmarie Gray, Barbara Jones, Yetta Rowland, Jim Carmichael, John Horsefall, Mike Sutton, Paul Stride, Helen Mead, Chris Johnson, Audrey Kirby, Julie Cork, Di Gritt, Sue Ormesher, Jackie Owen, David Andrews, Jackie Burnard, Philip Gordon, Rochelle Filda, Jane Mechlowitz, Karen Richman, Sue Stapley, Paula Walsh, Cathy Woodford, Karin Wimshurst, Stacia Briggs, Derek Fraser, Sandra Sutherland, Keith Stark, Maureen Morrison, Gill Cooper, Henry Trollope, Karen Collins, Robert Hurst, Hilary Lewis, Jane Harper, Isabel Coultas, Anne Smith, Norma Barker, Sandra Dean, Maggie Davis, Howard Leigh, Lisa Goldstein, Sandra Levinson, Richard Sears.

Many of those who helped with this book asked not to be mentioned but I am still very grateful to you all. If any names have been left out accidentally, I am sincerely sorry for any oversight on my part.

Preface

As I walked to the tube in my pre-pregnant days, I used to wonder why all the parents dropping their kids at school played 'I Will Survive' at top volume on their car stereos.

Two children later, having wrestled with the buggy, had numerous falls over the 'safety' gate, and torn my hair out trying to put together a travel cot, it suddenly became very clear. Misused baby products can damage both your health and your savings.

While there is no one piece of equipment that is perfect for every baby, there are certainly some that will make your life easier and save you money. *The Best Baby Buys Guide* selects a range of the best products, allowing you to make an informed choice that suits your own needs as well as your baby's.

'Great Value', 'Very Popular' and 'Luxury' buys (see p. 5) are based on the recommendations of families and retailers across Britain who have first-hand experience of what works and what does not. So, whether you are a new parent or an old hand, we believe that this guide is for you.

Good luck – you *will* survive!

Introduction

How this Book Can Save You Time and Money

If the road to hell is paved with good intentions, it has a hedgerow made of baby products! We set off for the shops, determined to buy the best for our babies, and end up dazed and in debt. Although there *are* some genuinely good-value, useful items around, it's difficult to distinguish the good from the bad.

Crucially, how do you know that you are buying items that are safe? An alarming number of fatalities arise from accidental misuse of highchairs, baby baths, buggies and (believe it or not) child safety equipment.

You need to be able to take your baby home safely, clothe him, feed him and give him somewhere appropriate to sleep. But, while you are dreaming of a blissful life with your forthcoming addition, some clever people in advertising have other plans.

They know that you are at a stage when you actually want to spend money so they shower you with leaflets and freebies. If a pregnant woman believed all the flyers and advertising material she was bombarded with, she would end up spending thousands of pounds that she could really do with later on.

Without babycare experience, how can you tell what is for you? Like most parents, you probably want to buy a buggy or pram but there are over a thousand models to choose from, ranging in price from £15 to £500. This is just the sort of problem *The Best Baby Buys Guide* can help you with.

Too many people are full of ghastly 'bad buy' stories. Don't follow in their footsteps. Before you start counting babygrows in your sleep, read this book. It will help you choose what is right for your needs and your budget.

Most importantly, if you want to concentrate on the development of your baby, rather than wasting time sourcing baby gear, *The Best Baby Buys Guide* is for you. Don't brave the hell that is the high street. Put your feet up and read this book. We have done the work for you. (You can even buy everything mail order – see pp. 7–8.)

Consumer Testing

Research was conducted in towns and cities across England, Scotland and Wales. Our team was chosen on the basis that they all had babies and excellent local knowledge and contacts. They were briefed to ask local baby goods shops and other families in the region about best and worst buys. Their views are based on personal experience. Prices given are believed to be accurate at the time of going to press.

Where products such as nappies needed to be tested by a variety of babies, this was supervised by the National Nursery Education Board (NNEB)-trained staff at Teddies Nurseries. This is the fastest-growing chain of day nurseries in England, with branches in 16 locations across the South and West of England. Teddies offers outstanding care and education for children aged three months to five years. They aim to promote confidence and independence in an environment that is welcoming and happy. Their staff are very special.

Safety

There is also the crucial issue of safety. You want to be sure that anything you buy is completely safe for your baby or toddler to use. For this reason many concerned manufacturers are members of the Baby Products Association.

The Baby Products Association (BPA)

The BPA represents a wide range of baby and nursery product suppliers. Their expert committees and working groups are instrumental in ensuring that Britain continues to have one of the safest baby equipment industries in the world.

BPA experts have looked at our recommendations to ensure that none of them contain known hazards.

Introduction

Your Views Count

If you have a 'best buy' that isn't included *we want to know* in time for the next edition, so please fill in the Reader's Report Form at the back of the book (freepost) or E-mail me at book4baby@aol.com. If you have a disaster we are equally interested...

How to Use this Book

This book is divided into three sections:

- Essential products for new babies.
- Optional products for new babies.
- Essentials for older babies.

Some readers may disagree with what we've categorised as optional but we've tried to go along with the majority opinion. Nursery monitors, for example, may be essential for some people – but not all. There is also an alphabetical contents list at the front of each section, and an exhaustive index at the back to help you find your dream baby product.

If you have already been shopping for baby equipment, you will know that there is a bewildering variety of goods available. We have designed each chapter to be a complete guide to each product as follows:

- A checklist highlights features (and possible hazards) to look out for when buying these products.
- A product table rounds off each chapter. This lists model, brand name, price and stockist, and includes comments from our researchers. Where relevant, we have flagged:

£ *Great Value Buy* – not necessarily the cheapest but a reasonably priced, good-quality product.

☺ *Very Popular Buy* – a product that wins a universal 'thumbs up' from users.

♛ *Luxury Buy* – a highly priced product that is worth considering if you have plenty of money and may make life that little bit easier.

Where to Shop
Chain Stores/Out-of-Town Retailers
It's worth bearing in mind that catalogue stores, such as Argos and Index, often have incredible bargains. And large branches of supermarket chains, such as Sainsburys and Tesco, have good-quality baby clothes at unbeatable prices. While you're there, look out for 'two for the price of one' offers on wipes, nappies, etc. Tesco Baby Club, Sainsbury's 0–5 Club and Safeway Baby Discount all offer shopping incentives to new mothers.

Babies 'R' Us (in Toys 'R' Us branches) have a computerised 'Baby Gift List' service, allowing you to list your favourite items for your loving family and friends to go in and buy.

Specialist Baby Shops
Independent shops may look out of keeping with your hip, new parent image but the prices may be more competitive than you realise – some offer a 'never knowingly undersold' guarantee. And even in a small shop there are usually a larger variety of products for sale. (Multiples tend to carry fewer lines that they know they can shift quickly.) Also, the smaller shops are geared up to place special orders, so you can get what you really want, rather than settling for what happens to be on display.

> Never leave any shop without being perfectly clear how to use what you've bought. If a badly assembled buggy is going to collapse you can be sure that it will happen in the middle of the road.

The Nippers Chain
These are nursery shops operating from barns on farms. They offer easy parking, good prices (as overheads are minimal) and, often, a good variety of second-hand equipment. They will not sell second-hand car seats or equipment that does not conform to current standards. There are branches in Hildenborough (Tel: 01732 838333); Canterbury (Tel: 01227 832006); Milton Keynes (Tel: 01908 504506);

Introduction

Colchester (Tel: 01787 228000); Chessington (Tel: 0181 398 3114); Rugby (Tel: 01926 633100); Worcester (Tel: 01386 750888) and Royston (Tel: 01223 207071). Opening hours may vary so ring before you set off.

Mail Order

If you don't have the time or the inclination to visit the high street, or you don't have easy access to shops, you can order everything you need from catalogues.

However, a word of warning: we ordered mail order catalogues at two different times of the year to see how this altered the response time. As a general rule we discovered that if you order when the catalogue has just been launched, you tend to receive an excellent service and the full choice of goods is available – although they may be delivered in dribs and drabs.

But if you ring for a catalogue towards the end of the season, it may not arrive at all, although in many cases we must have been added to a mailing list for new ones suddenly turned up, unrequested, many weeks later.

Mail order companies are listed throughout the book under the various product categories but, generally, it's worth having the following catalogues to hand:

Shop	Catalogue	Telephone
Boots	*Mother and Baby at Home Catalogue*	0845 840 1000
Mothercare	*Newborn to Toddler Catalogue*	01923 240365 (Avoid ringing at peak times)
Tesco	*Baby and Toddler Catalogue*	0345 024024

For Londoners and people who live in Richmond, Surrey:

Trotters/Nappy Express	Next-day delivery for competitively priced nappies, foods and household items. Free delivery.	Tel: 0181 368 4040 Ansaphone and fax orders: 0181 368 0132

For pregnant women who need both maternity wear and baby goods:

Blooming Marvellous	Catalogues: 0181 391 4822; Orders: 0181 391 0338
JoJo Maman Bébé	Catalogues: 0171 352 5156; Orders: 0171 351 4112

There are a number of catalogues whose product range is based on quality and innovation rather than budgetary considerations. One group of London mothers were uniformly lavish in their praise of the Great Little Trading Company (Tel: 0990 673008). This company offers a range of unusual and interesting baby products delivered within five working days. They import quite a few goods from the US which are tricky to find in other stores.

Internet
A number of companies allow you to order via the World Wide Web. This is particularly useful if you want an American product that is hard to track down over here. (You will have to pay tax on goods ordered from abroad.) If you fancy some US-style parenting advice, check out the Pampers Parenting Institute on www.Pampers.com. An excellent British site is http://www.ukmums.co.uk – well worth a visit. Also of interest is www.babyworld.com, another UK site.

We found it difficult to track relevant companies down using a standard search engine such as Yahoo. Where we have found web sites, we have listed them with telephone and fax numbers.

Free Baby Equipment
Look out for the competitions and special offers in pregnancy and baby magazines. We came across an ecstatic mother who had won an expensive highchair through a reader offer.

Best-selling monthly titles that you may enjoy reading – even if you don't win anything – include *Baby*, *Our Baby*, *Prima Baby*, *Practical Parenting*, *Mother and Baby*, *Junior* and *M*.

Buying Second-Hand Baby Equipment

A lot of parents and grandparents feel that 'only new will do' for their little miracle. But a pram, for instance, is only in use for around six months and can easily cost £300. So it's worth considering a second-hand model, which will leave you more to spend on essentials such as nappies. However, *if in doubt, buy new*. You cannot afford to take risks with your baby's safety.

Where to Shop
Only buy well-maintained second-hand equipment from a reliable source. Around one-third of the nursery equipment in use is second-hand but that does not mean that it is all either safe or suitable.

Car boot sales and newspaper ads placed by individuals should be treated with caution.

'Nearly New' Shops
'Nearly new' baby equipment shops often have a fast turnover of stock, so it is worth leaving them a list of the products you are looking for – the earlier into your pregnancy you can do this, the better. Some baby equipment shops have a second-hand goods section, e.g. the Nippers chain (see pp. 6–7). The advantages of buying from a reputable second-hand shop are that:

- Even if equipment is virtually unused, it will still cost less than the new version.
- They will not knowingly supply anything dangerous.

Buyer Beware
Falls
When using equipment that is high (like a highchair or pram), a five-point harness should prevent falls. Make sure that products have no ledges, steps or footholds that might tempt a baby to climb high and fall over or destabilise equipment.

Foreign Goods
Be particularly careful if you are considering goods bought overseas. As with second-hand goods, these do not have to meet any safety standards. Look out for BS or EN labels which show that an item complies with either British or European standards (see p. 12).

Faulty Locks
A baby may be crushed by a piece of equipment collapsing with him inside it. So check that all locks work efficiently

and cannot come undone while in use. Toddlers may also fiddle with equipment when your back is turned. So if a product has a storage lock when not in use (e.g. a fold-up pushchair or highchair), it must work.

Loose Fittings
Check every moving part. If they move awkwardly or bits come off that shouldn't, do not buy. Your child might put a loose fitting in his mouth and choke on it. Similarly, he could suffocate if he accidentally has loose plastic pressed against his mouth and nose at the same time. Check loose covers to ensure that this cannot happen.

Missing Parts
If a product does not come with all its fittings, be sure that you can replace these easily before you buy. If not, don't. The item's accompanying instruction leaflet should detail exactly what comes with it.

No Instructions
Be wary if the instruction leaflet is missing. Some equipment is virtually impossible to assemble without it.

Old Paint and Varnish
If you are considering using an old piece of equipment without a BS number that has peeling paint or flaking varnish, see if you can strip it off and redo the finish with a non-toxic product before using it. Your baby could poison himself otherwise. The paint may be dangerous if it is not made to BS or EN standards

Stability
Check that an item is stable by lifting it slightly and seeing if it drops back to its original position.

Tears and Splits
If stuffing is seeping through a split in a seat, your child may be tempted to put this in his mouth. This could easily present a choking hazard. If the seat covers hard or sharp edges, splits in the fabric could uncover these and could bruise or

cut the baby. Run your hands along all edges and surfaces to make sure that they are smooth.

Traps
Use a pencil to poke into any hole which may tempt small fingers. Move adjustable parts to see if they maim or cut the pencil and then imagine what these could do to curious fingers. Make sure that there is no hole large enough to trap limbs or a head.

> ## Products that You Should Never Buy Second-Hand
> - Mattresses – could harbour bugs, mould, etc.
> - Car seats – could have been weakened in an accident. It is usually impossible to assess by inspection if this is the case.

Generally speaking, the simpler the product, the fewer things there are to go wrong. Look out for items that you will only use for a few months. They must be very clean (this is usually a sign of good maintenance) and you must feel confident that you can clean them easily yourself. Don't buy anything too old, as you may not be able to get spare parts when you need them.

To give you an idea of the possible savings to be made, here are four examples of products bought new and second-hand. Generally, second-hand goods seem to be marked at roughly half the price they would retail at new, but this depends on the condition they are in. Retailers seem to set prices according to the age, wear and tear and cleanliness of the goods.

Product	Price When New (approx)	Product Details on Pages	Price Second-hand
Baby carrier	£20–£45	157–159	£5–£20
Swinging chair	£70–£90	163	£35
Travel cot	£60–£80	203–204	£15–£25 (You will need to buy a new mattress)

Product	Price When New (approx)	Product Details on Pages	Price Second-hand
Bouncer (doorframe)	£40	152–153	£15

British and European Standards for Baby Products

There are over 50 British Standards for specific baby products, in addition to numerous standards governing general applications such as labelling and wiring. Each standard is regularly examined by the British Standards Institute (BSI) and revised when necessary.

European (EN) standards, developed by the Comité Européen de Normalisation in Brussels, are increasingly beginning to replace British ones. The Baby Products Association has representatives on all relevant committees and 30 new standards are currently under development, with some already published.

Although Britain has an excellent international reputation for safety, guidelines for testing are being tightened up even further. Ultimately, you must decide if you think something does not look as solid or as safe as you would wish. The BS/EN mark should be used as a guide only. If there is no mark at all – be wary. It should not be for sale.

Preparing for Twins and Triplets

It's reckoned that it takes 197 hours a week to care for triplets but there are only 168 hours available. Imagine having to sterilise 18 bottles in one go and you have an idea of the chores in store.

But, as one mother wrote of her twins, 'Nothing beats a hug from two little pairs of arms.' So here are a few tips to give you more time for hugs and minimise the time you spend on the more mundane aspects.

Before You Buy Anything...
Join Tamba, The Twins and Multiple Births Association (Tel: 0870 121 4000). They will put you in touch with your local

Twins Club which should prove to be a great source of second-hand equipment and first-hand experience.

> **Crucial Kit**
> - Washing machine and a separate tumble-dryer.
> - Two kettles.
> - A delivery service or a neighbour who will help out with the shopping as it can prove difficult to get out of the house – even for essentials.
> - Telephone answer machine or BT callminder system costing about £6 a quarter (Tel: 0800 252599).

Twins or Triplets Need their Own:

- *Bouncy chairs (cheaper versions – see p. 162) or a playpen to share*. These will enable you to put them down safely when the doorbell goes or you need to pick up the phone.
- *Cots (eventually) (see below, pp. 14–15, and pp. 69–74).*
- *Highchairs (see pp. 217–223)*. Mothers preferred cube versions as these become low tables and chairs which are useful later on. Tesco Direct have a three-in-one cube for £39.99.
- *Potties (see pp. 224–227)*. They definitely need their own, otherwise you will have to deal with overflow problems.

Travel
Buggies

- For a heavy-duty buggy for infant twins many mothers liked the Emmaljunga Twin 'Grizzly' stroller (£299) which should fit through most front doors.
- Preferred lighter-weight models are the two Maclaren twin buggies – the Duette (£159) and the Mistral Duo (£129) – and the Mamas and Papas Twin Micro Coperto (£210).
- Parents of triplets have very little choice in the buggy line and you will incur huge expenses by having a twin buggy adapted for triplets over six months. The cheapest option we could find for triplets of six months plus was Gordon's triple lightweight buggy for £235 (Tel: 0161 740 9979).
- Up to six months, many triplets' parents use a bench-seat twin (Bébé Confort or Mothercare £199) with three harnesses, or put two in a buggy and carry one in a sling.

Car Seats

- The Britax Rock-a-Tot (£59.99) was hugely liked by parents for two reasons. Firstly it seemed to offer good support to low-birthweight babies. Secondly, it was useful as a rocking chair in the home. You can rock one baby with your foot while you cuddle or feed the other.

Travel Highchairs
- If you are planning to take them out to eat, you can buy soft roll-up seats that attach to most chairs and will fit into your changing bag from Boots (£14.99).

Round the House
Safety Gadgets
- Twins and triplets seem extra-good at getting round safety devices ('One pushes while the other pulls' was one parent's explanation), so you will need to think carefully about safety. Most parents thought that door slam stoppers (£3.99 for two at most nursery outlets) were an essential buy. Plug covers and other apparently useful items were swiftly removed by some crafty pairs.

Sleeping
- Most parents preferred putting their babies straight into cot beds in their own room. These last longer than a cot and can be incredibly good value.
- One mother put her infant twins into adjacent Moses baskets in her own room, with a mobile fixed on the side of one basket so that both twins could watch it.

Changing
- As time is short, all the parents we spoke to used disposable nappies.
- All parents said a rucksack-style changing bag was essential so that you can carry it on your back while your hands are free to deal with the babies.

Dressing
- You don't need two or three of everything. Just have plenty of neutral babygrows and vests that they can all wear.

Bottle Feeding
- It is easier to make up multiple feeds in one large jug rather than messing around with individual bottles.
- Silicone teats are much harder-wearing.

- A large-capacity steam steriliser that only takes nine minutes is vital. A number of parents had two of these. With these, you can avoid spending time rinsing sterilising solution off endless bottles and teats.

Equipping Your Home for a Special Needs Baby
Grants

First try Social Services. If they cannot help you with particular items, the reference section of your library should have a book called *Grants for Individuals in Need*. If you look up the relevant sections (specific disabilities, aid for children, and the area you live in), you should get an idea of the available options.

The Disabled Living Foundation (Equipment helpline: 0870 603 9177; Minicom: 0870 603 9176) can send you a leaflet on raising funds.

Fact Sheets

The Disabled Living Foundation will also send up to three sets of fact sheets, free of charge, to disabled people and their carers. Statutory services, health professionals and organisations are required to pay £2.50 per copy.

Titles include: 'Choosing Children's Daily Living Equipment', 'Choosing Children's Play Equipment' and 'Choosing Children's Mobility Equipment'.

Domestic Alterations

If you think you will need to alter your home to accommodate the needs of your baby, information and advice are available from the Centre for Accessible Environments (CAE), Nutmeg House, 60 Gainsford Street, London SE1 2NY (Tel: 0171 357 8182). The Centre provides publications and access to a database of building professionals, architects, surveyors, etc, who are experienced in building and structural alterations to accommodate the needs of disabled people.

Section 1: The Bare Necessities

Baby Clothes

Why do so many of us feel the need to dress our children as unidentified furry objects? In front of me are catalogues selling everyday clothes in which babies are dressed as numerous breeds of dog, a teddy and even a cuddly pumpkin.

I know there is a lot wrong with looking like a baby – double chin, bald spot, no cheekbones, etc, etc – but surely we should allow our infants to be young gracefully. Why not put them in the ultimate minimalist chic – the Tesco white cotton bodysuit (£2.50 for two)?

It may be hard to resist the temptation but it really isn't worth buying loads of expensive clothes for a newborn baby. One mother commented, 'I realised how much I was wasting on clothes when, every few weeks, I kept having to buy more. Now I get all "outfits" at charity or nearly new shops. It's fantastic – they are hardly worn "labels" at a fraction of the price.'

What you really need are clothes that are comfortable, safe and an appropriate weight for the time of year. From a carer's point of view, you want baby clothes that are stretchy, washable and have easy nappy access. 'I regretted everything I bought that lacked poppers at the crotch,' said one mother. Some parents rate natural fibres as equally important.

A baby will be uncomfortable if his clothes are tight, wrinkly, rough, lumpy or push into his skin. So look for soft, good-quality garments.

Shopping List
- Six to eight stretchsuits.
- Six vests.
- Two cardigans or sweatshirts.

- Three bibs.
- Two pairs socks.
- *Summer babies* – a light jacket and sun hat.
- *Winter babies* – warm hat, mittens, snowsuit.

Checklist
Seams

- There should be no coarse internal seams. Be particularly finicky about appliquéd designs – is there scratchy stitching on the inside?
- Remember that your baby will spend a large amount of his day on his back. For this reason you should go for clothes that open at the front so that he's not lying on a seam.
- Check that the seams are thoroughly bound with thread so they are unable to fray with repeated washing.

Necklines

- Check that the neckline isn't too tight – babies hate having clothes pulled on over their faces.
- Instead look for envelope necks or necks with poppers at the side so that they can be opened wide to slip over your baby's head.

Nappy Access

- For small babies, look for clothes that offer quick access to the bottom so a nappy can be changed without taking everything off. You do not want to slip soiled garments over your baby's face.
- Look for poppers at the crotch.

Easy-Care Garments

- Endearing little habits, such as drooling, projectile vomiting and exploding nappies, mean that some babies go through a number of outfits in a day. So clothes must be able to go in the washing machine on a regularly used cycle.
- Ideally you want clothes that need minimal ironing.

Baby Clothes

- Avoid biological washing powders and fabric conditioners as they could irritate your baby's skin.
- Never buy 'dry-clean only' garments.

Fabrics
- You are generally given a choice between 100% cotton and a cotton/polyester mix. Polycotton has two advantages: it is less likely to shrink in the wash and it needs minimal ironing. We found 100% cotton jersey equally user-friendly.
- If you buy cheap garments of uncertain origin (e.g. from a market stall) you may find that they shrink or become rough to the touch.

Hidden Dangers
- Clothes must not restrict the circulation. Watch out for elasticated wrist and ankle holes that leave red marks.
- Loose threads, buttons, stray pins in home-made garments, could catch a little finger or toe. Also watch out for the wide weave of a home-knitted cardigan or a label that is sewn on in a loop (cut these at the base) as a finger caught in these could also prove painful at the best and dangerous at worst.
- Be wary of ribbons or ties that could prove a risk of strangulation or that your baby might be tempted to suck and possibly choke on. Ribbons or ties should usually be no longer than 220mm or about 9 inches.

Stretchsuits/Sleepsuits/Babygrows
- These are the all-in-one outfits worn day and night by most small babies.
- As soon as your baby's feet appear constricted by the stretchsuit, put it away – or cut the feet off the garment and hem the bottoms.

Gowns
- Gowns are great for speedy nappy changes. So if you are expecting twins or more, these may be preferable to stretchsuits.

- Some come with drawstring bottoms to stop them riding up.

Vests/Bodysuits
These come in three designs:

- Wrapovers which you tie with a bow (pretty but fiddly).
- Vests which are a tiny version of the adult garment (these may ride up).
- Bodysuits with an envelope neckline and poppers at the crotch to ensure a snug fit (the best).

Cardigans/Sweatshirts
- Sweatshirts with buttons on the shoulder are easier to put on and take off.

Mittens
- Buy mittens. Don't even consider gloves. Trying to get them onto little fingers in the freezing cold is like eating spaghetti without cutlery.
- Some mittens come on a string that you thread through the coat arms. Some people think that this is a strangulation risk but others think the risk is minimal and worth taking so as not to lose the mittens. Metal clips to secure gloves and mittens to the sleeve are available by mail order – JoJo (Tel: 0171 351 4112) sell two pairs for £4.99.

Foot Protection
- Knitted bootees are difficult to keep on. Go for one-size stretchy socks (in stock at Baby Gap and Hennes as we went to press) or padded, elasticated bootees.
- If you need some dainty baby shoes to go with a special outfit and money is no object, Nursery Emporium (Mail order: 01249 811310) supply handmade baby shoes in gingham or broderie anglaise fabric (£24 plus p&p).

Snowsuits
- These all-in-one suits, usually made of showerproof fabric, are only appropriate for a new baby if you are continuously carrying him in and out of the car in a car

seat. Otherwise you do not need one until he is old enough to travel round town sitting in a stroller. (If your baby goes out in a pram, he should have sufficient warmth and protection if he wears a hat and is covered with blankets and a showerproof cover.)
- When you do buy a snowsuit, make sure it's showerproof.
- It should also have a hood for additional protection (to be used in conjunction with a hat) when there is a bitter wind.
- It must be fully machine-washable.
- Some snowsuits have mittens and bootees on poppers – an excellent way to reduce the lost sock and lost mitten count.

Pyjamas
- These are a very optional extra but some parents are mad keen to put their 12-month-old sons into traditional PJs.
- The best-value traditional selection we could find was that offered by FIG. Their designs come in 100% cotton and range from the staid to the stunning (£16 a pair for all children's sizes). They also supply nighties. They can be contacted on Tel: 01728 660551; or E-mail: chappel@btinternet.com.

Traditional Babywear
- If you want a hand-made cardigan or shawl, Pride and Joy are a mother-and-daughter team in Scotland who produce a range of knitted woollens for small babies. Most items cost £15 or £16. Telephone for a catalogue: 01721 752686.
- Clair de Lune have a range of christening wear. Telephone for a catalogue and a list of local stockists: 0161 283 4476/7.

Sizes
- It is usual to buy clothes a size larger than your baby (e.g. for a one-month-old buy a three-month size).
- European brands' equivalent sizes tend to come up smaller.

- For outerwear, buy one size larger than the rest of your baby's clothes so that you can fit them all underneath.
- The following table is a rough guide to sizes.

Age	Height	Weight
Early baby	Up to 50cm	Up to 3.5kg
Newborn	50–56cm	Up to 4.5kg
0–3 months	56–62cm	Up to 6.5kg
3–6 months	62–68cm	Up to 8kg
6–9 months	68–74cm	Up to 9kg
9–12 months	74–80cm	Up to 10.5kg
12–18 months	80–86cm	Up to 12kg
18–24 months	86–92cm	–

Hangers for Baby Clothes

As soon as the little blue line appears, start collecting suitable hangers. Marks & Spencer lingerie and women's trouser hangers with adjustable clips are good. Put a bit of tissue paper between the clip and the garment to prevent marks. Otherwise, try mail order companies – Blooming Marvellous (Tel: 0191 391 4822) sell a pack of 10 for £2.99 (children's size). Padded versions for special outfits are sold by Nursery Emporium and Urchin (Tel: 01672 871515).

Product Table

What we looked for:

- Ease of putting on.
- Fit.
- Comfort.
- Softness.
- Value for money.
- How well they washed.

Clothes for Newborns

Stockists	Products
Adams	100% cotton sleepsuits (£8.99 for two); pack of two bodysuits (from £3.99).
Asda	Three white cotton bodysuits (£9.99).
Baby Gap	If you are travelling to the US, pay Gap a visit as prices are lower than in UK stores. If you win the lottery, this is where to spend it.
Blooming Marvellous (Mail order: 0181 391 0338)	Small but fully co-ordinating selection in 100% cotton or cotton jersey. Prices from £6.99 for an animal print short-sleeved vest.
Boots	Extensive range in 100% cotton that can all be seen and ordered into your local shop via the *Your Baby and You* catalogue. Pack of two bodysuits (from £6); pack of two decorated sleepsuits (from £10).
BHS	Pack of three white sleepsuits (£9); pack of two bodysuits (£5.50).
Hennes	Trendy outfits for under £10. Also basics such as: two long-sleeved vests (£5.99); All in One (£12.99); two pairs of stretchy terry stay-on socks (£1.50).
John Lewis	Two Jonelle-brand vests (£3.45); two stretchsuits (£7.95); padders (£5.95).
JoJo (Mail order: 0171 351 4112)	If you can't bear pure white, JoJo do a 100% cotton starter pack with a cow appliqué for £21.99. This includes two sleepsuits, two short-sleeved bodysuits and two pop-over bibs. Or, if buying separately, two cow sleepsuits (£12.99); two bodysuits (vests), short-sleeved (£6.99), all 100% cotton.
Marks & Spencer ☺	Four sleepsuits (£16); four short-sleeved bodysuits (£9); three long-sleeved bodysuits (£9).
Mothercare (Mail order: 01923 240365)	100% cotton range for newborns and small babies includes pack of three white bodysuits (£4.50); pack of three white sleepsuits (£9). For a full range visit your local store or use the mail order catalogue.

Clothes for Newborns (continued)

Stockists	Products
NCT (Mail order: 0141 636 0600)	NCT (National Childbirth Trust) do a range of 100% cotton co-ordinating nightshirts for parents (from £17.95) to match their baby's long-sleeved vest (£5.25).
Next (Mail order: 0345 100500)	Good choice of complete outfits under £20, available through local branches or mail order. The catalogue costs a non-refundable £3 but it contains a wide range of family clothing and home furnishings.
Petit Bateau (Mail order plus delivery charge from Rachel Riley: 0171 259 5969). Also available from all smart baby shops.	Wonderful-quality, beautiful designs but only worthwhile if you are planning a number of babies. These wash perfectly and last indefinitely. Long-sleeved bodysuit, blue or pink (£14); polo collar bodysuit (£11); lace collar bodysuit (£16). Their wrapover vests with a little bow are the only ones of this type that seem to stay put. They were highly recommended by a mother whose baby hated envelope-neck vests being lowered over his head.
Tesco (Orders: 0345 024024)	If you're bored with shopping for your baby but he still hasn't appeared, the answer is the Tesco Hospital Pack (£29.99). This includes bodysuits, sleepsuits, changing bag, breast pads, nappies, etc. Otherwise: pack of two vests (£3); two sleepsuits (£7), all 100% cotton.
Woolworths (Ladybird)	100% cotton: three-pack of sleepsuits (£9.99); three-pack of bodysuits (£4.99). Amazing baby bargains include: jogpants (£3.99), T-shirts (£1.99) and denim dungarees (£7.99).

Clothes for Premature Babies

If the Special Care Baby Unit will lend you some, don't buy these as you will be amazed how quickly your baby grows.

These have not been tested, but if you need some in a hurry...

Premature Baby Clothes

Stockists	Products
Incubaby	Clothes with openings for tubes and probes for babies in incubators. You have to order these by visiting your local nursery shop and choosing from the brochure. They place the order and 48-hour delivery is guaranteed. Otherwise orders are taken via the Internet.
Babycare, Cherish Dollycare	Sister ranges to Incubaby so order from brochure as above. For babies of under 3kg.
Tiddlywinks (Mail order: 01274 561751)	For babies of 1kg+. Prices from £2 for a vest.
Tiny Trends (Mail order: 01202 523060)	For babies of 1.5kg+. They include outfits for babies in incubators that allow for tubes and probes. Babygrows £4.55 each.
Small Wonder (Mail order: 0181 886 1956)	For babies of 1.5–3.5kg. A pack of three babygrows costs £13.99.

Clothes for Crawlers and Toddlers

All the high-street brands mentioned on pp. 25–26 have ranges that cover this age group.

If you are looking for some medium-priced mail-order solutions, check out the following:

Crawler and Toddler Clothes

Catalogue	Products
Cotton Moon (Orders: 0181 305 0012)	Trousers (£15.95); roll-neck sweatshirt (£8.95).
Mini Boden (Orders: 0181 453 1535)	Trousers (£16); roll-neck sweatshirt (£13).

Crawler and Toddler Clothes (continued)

Catalogue	Products
Trotters Direct (Orders: 0990 331188)	Trousers (£21.99); sweatshirts (£9.99). Also stock Petit Bateau underwear for children.
Verbaudet (Orders: 0500 012345)	Trousers (£13.99); roll-neck sweatshirt – small sizes (£6.99).

£

Baths

You can get by without a baby bath for new babies. Instead you can use a basin of water and a towel. Most people who buy a baby bath use it for only a few weeks until they feel confident using the standard bath for their baby.

However, there are two reasons to consider some sort of bathing aid. Firstly, if your back is too weak to bend over a bath tub, a baby bath allows you to wash your baby without stooping forward. Secondly, your baby may tend to slide from your grasp once he's covered in soap. A bath or a baby bathing support (see pp. 30–31) will minimise this.

Be careful if you buy a cheap, unbranded baby bath – it may fold under the weight of the water.

Many shops sell baths packaged with 'gifts' inside. Ignore these as you may end up paying for a useless bath and pointless products. A top and tail bowl, for instance, is not essential – any bowl will do.

Some mothers we interviewed enjoyed sharing their own bath with their baby. If you're tempted to follow suit but don't want your baby to metamorphose into a boiled prawn, remember to keep the water lukewarm. Always check the water with your elbow to ensure it's not too hot, and never place the baby in the bath first before you run the water, as it may be hotter than you expect.

For babies who can sit up, a non-slip bath mat will prevent 'slippery baby syndrome'. If your older baby hates having his face near the water, you may want to buy a bath ring (a circular seat on suction cups that attach to the base of the bath). This should keep your baby upright while you wash him. But never treat a bath ring as a safety aid. You must *never* leave your baby alone in the bath – even if it's just for a moment to answer the telephone or door.

Shopping List
- Baby bath plus stand, or bath support for use in standard bath.
- Non-slip bath mat (don't waste money on a 'baby' one – a full-sized one costs £1 or so more but lasts longer).
- Towel (for baby's sole use).
- Baby toiletries of your choice (e.g. bubble bath or soap, sponge, shampoo).
- Milk-teeth toothpaste and infant tooth brush (see pp. 244–247).
- Bath ring (for babies of six months plus).

Checklist
Traditional Baby Bath
- This is a plastic container for use in the bath or on a stand.
- It should have a rounded end so that it slots under the tap for easy filling.
- It also needs a plug hole so you don't have to lift it for emptying when it's full of water.
- Some people buy a new washing-up bowl instead of a baby bath, as this is inexpensive and can be put to good use afterwards. For hygiene purposes, don't use it for anything else while it is in use as a bath.

Bath that Slots on Top of Your Bath
- These are large but easy to use – as long as they fit onto your bath. (Measure your bath before you buy one and check that it fits before you unwrap it.)
- Also check that the baby bath has a plug hole, for easy emptying.

Tummy Tub
- This bucket-like bath is less unwieldy than a traditional baby bath and requires less water to fill it than a standard bath.

Bath Support
- If you want some help but don't fancy having your bath tub colonised by a vast piece of plastic, a bath support is

ideal. These are small seats or nests that go straight into the bath. They come in a variety of materials, ranging from foam to moulded plastic.
- If you are trying to choose between a bath and a bath support, the support is smaller, cheaper and does the job perfectly.

Bath Ring
- This is for older babies who can sit up unaided – and it must never be used as a safety aid. The ring keeps your baby sitting upright in the bath while you wash him.
- As a general rule, you may find it difficult to get a larger baby in and out.

Baby Bath Stand
- This should be treated as a very optional extra. This is a foldaway stand that holds a baby bath at waist height. It is supposed to be useful for women with bad backs. But, as you still have to lift a bath full of water on and off the stand, I don't see the logic of this.
- If you are worried about bending over a bath, you can use a baby bath that slots on top of the bath. You kneel beside the bath to use one of these.
- Alternatively, you can buy a changing unit with an integral bath (see pp. 65–68) – if you can find a way of filling the bath without lugging water around.

Non-Slip Bath Mats
- These are essential for babies not using a baby bath. They limit sliding and bumping on the bottom of the bath and so make it far easier to bathe your baby.
- People who bought traditional baby baths also liked them, as they offer a better surface to hold the baby bath in place.

Product Table

What we looked for:

- Ease of use.
- Value for money.

Baths for New Babies

Brand and Price	Stockists	Comments
Warning: Whatever you choose never be tempted to leave your baby alone in the water.		
Traditional Baby Baths		
Boots Baby Bath (£14.49)	Boots	This has no plug hole and may not fit right under the taps in your bath. It does have slots in the side for easy carrying. But it's expensive compared to competition.
Bath Supports		
Bettacare Batheasy (£8.99) £	John Lewis, independent retailers	Flannel deckchair on wire frame, to be used in a standard bath. Cheap, small, easy to clean. Hugely popular.
Cheeky Rascals Baby Bath Seat (£14.95) ♛	Cheeky Rascals (Mail order: 01428 682488)	Need to fill bath quite high to stop baby getting cold but a good solid product. 'I felt really confident with this' was a common response.
Eezi Sponge Support (£5.99)	Mothercare, John Lewis, independent retailers	Foam support that sits in standard bath. Like all damp foam, this can go smelly with age. The jury was divided on this, some found it slipped around – others couldn't have lived without it.
Baths That Fit on Top of Your Own		
Supabath (£18)	Mothercare (and Mothercare mail order, Tel: 01923 240365)	Contoured to help support a baby. Features an integral soap dish and plug. Excellent.
Eezi Bath (£16) ☺	John Lewis, independent retailers	Rectangular rigid plastic bath designed to sit across your bath. Has plug hole. Good alternative to Mothercare's Supabath.

Baths for New Babies (continued)

Brand and Price	Stockists	Comments
Unusual Models		
Tummy Tub (£15.99)	John Lewis, Baby Warehouse mail order (see below)	Ideal if you want a stand-alone bath, as its bucket-shape uses less water than other types so it's lighter to carry around. May seem odd to us but it is the top seller in Europe.
2-In-1 Infant/Toddler Tub (£16.99)	The Baby Warehouse (Mail order: 0181 852 1122)	Designed for both babies and toddlers although toddlers may find it restricting and not such fun as a full-size bath. Contains an inner shell to keep baby's head and shoulders clear of the water.
Tomy Portable Soft Bath (£9.95)	John Lewis	Inflatable, for easy travel and storage. The lungs of an opera singer and the patience of a saint would be handy but Tomy report massive sales. They think it's particularly popular for people travelling. It weighs next to nothing.
Bath Seats for Older Babies		
Swivel Bath Seat Safety First (£12.99)	Tel: 0181 236 0707 for stockists	Well-made design with good back support. Easy to operate, allowing seat to be turned and locked at any point.

Bath Products

It's hard enough having to wash a baby, let alone juggle him with bottles full of bubble bath. Although it may enhance your bathroom decor to have loads of baby products, you really don't need that many. The absolute maximum required by most parents is soap or baby bath, with baby shampoo as an optional extra. Babies with dry skin may benefit from a post-wash application of baby lotion.

Checklist
Soap and Bubble Bath

- All supermarkets and major chemists sell own-brand bath products for babies. If you find that these dry your baby's skin, try either Infaderm or Oilatum.
- Some people swear by putting a few drops of olive oil in the bath water or massaging almond oil (from pharmacy counters) into the skin.
- Johnson & Johnson products were top of most people's list. Boots and Sainsbury's also came out very well in our tests. Sainsbury's Moisturising Baby Bath with Baby Oil (£1.79 for 500ml) 'left skin silky smooth'.

Sponges (or Cotton Wool Pads or a Flannel)

- Be sure that you, not your baby, are in charge of the sponge. Some babies try to chew them.
- Embossed cotton wool pads may be better when washing small babies. Normal cotton wool tends to disintegrate in strands on their bodies.

Towels

- You don't need a special type of towel. For hygiene purposes ensure that your baby's towel is not shared with anyone else.

Bath Products

Shampoo

- All the family can use baby shampoo but do check the 'fragrance' before you buy.
- Baby shampoos tend to be gentler than normal shampoos and some have a 'no tears' formula. Without this, hair washing can become the most dreaded form of water combat since the Armada. We therefore rate Johnsons 'No More Tears' Baby Shampoo (£1.25 for 200ml), Boots Hypo-Allergenic No Tears Baby Shampoo (£1.25 for 250ml), Sainsbury No Tears (£1.09 for 300ml) and Tesco Baby Shampoo (99p for 300ml – a real bargain, if you like the perfume).

Optional Extras

- Baby lotion, baby oil, cotton buds. Sainsbury's Baby Lotion (£1.09 for 300ml) was 'excellent – left skin soft and smooth but not greasy'.
- Inflatable tap covers to stop older babies hurting themselves on the edge of a tap. See table on p. 234.

Talcum Powder

- If using talcum powder, you should be careful not to get any near your baby's nose and mouth because of the risk of choking.
- Put a little powder on some cotton wool and carefully apply where needed.

Bath Temperature Thermometers

- You really do not need one of these.
- When you run the bath, just run the cold water, turn off the tap, mix in some hot water, and turn off the tap. Finish off with a little cold water and then test with your elbow to ensure that it is not too hot.
- If the hot water comes out of your taps scalding, turn down the thermostat. This will avoid accidents and save money on your heating bills. If you can't, a plumber can fit a device to regulate the heat on the bath tap.

Bath Toys

- Bath toys certainly aren't essential but they can make bathtime a lot more fun (see p. 196). They may also help you tempt reluctant bathers into the water.

Bottle Feeding

You wander into Mothercare, see a display of bottles and think, 'I need those.' What you don't realise is that these innocuous little objects can be the source of as much joy, relief, grief, pain, frustration and irritation as England's performance in the World Cup.

Some bottles leak; some are impossible to clean; and others cannot stand vertical with a feed inside them. A few people cannot get on with standard shaped bottles and find themselves pouring scalding formula over their hands on a regular basis – hardly the ultimate in skincare treatments. But there is immense satisfaction in finding a feeding system that appeals to a previously uninterested feeder.

All this drama from one little bottle . . .

Shopping List
- Six bottles.
- Eight slow-flow teats (for smaller babies), medium to fast-flow for larger babies.
- Bottle brush/teat brush.
- Steriliser (see pp. 43–47).
- *For bottle feeding on the move consider*: Umix feeding system, disposable bottles, bottle carrier, formula storage containers.

Breastfeeding is considered the better option in the early months, as it is a tailor-made diet that also benefits your baby's immune system. And it's free. However, most mothers succumb to the lure of formula at some point.

When you do, follow the instructions for making up formula carefully, and always buy the right formula for your baby's age – otherwise it could prove too rich for his immature system. You should never add anything to the formula unless specified by your doctor.

Note: If your baby has been under medical supervision, you may qualify for formula on prescription.

Bottle Checklist
Capacity
- The regular size is 250ml.
- You may want some smaller bottles for drinks between feeds but these are a short-term luxury as most babies take up to 225ml by the time they hit four months.

Standard Bottles
- These classic, narrow cylindrical bottles (that you can get from every baby shop) will fit a range of teats.
- Undecorated ones are usually the cheapest and some sterilisers can do eight of these at one go. However, the narrow neck makes them tricky to fill.

Wide-Neck Bottles
- These shorter, stubbier models, pioneered by Avent, take the same quantity of milk as standard bottles.
- With the exception of the Tommee Tippee wide-neck range, they only take silicone teats.
- They are the easiest to fill and clean.

Shaped Bottles
- These bottles, shaped like a stretched Polo mint with a hole in the middle, help older babies grip the bottle and feed themselves.
- However, shaped bottles are hard to clean and difficult to use with formula, as it is tricky to mix thoroughly, so you might want to mix the formula in a jug first.

Disposable Bottle Systems
- These are good for short holidays because you do not need to sterilise the bottles. Instead, you buy disposable sterilised bags that fit into a bottle-shaped holder.
- Some people use these instead of normal bottles because they believe that the way the bags contract, as the baby sucks, ensures that no air is taken in with the feed, thus relieving colic.

- At around £4 for 10 pre-sterilised bags and one teat, this is expensive for daily use. The teats are non-disposable and will need to be cleaned and sterilised. For long-term use, Avent offer a system including 80 bags and a storage box/steriliser (available from Boots mail order, £19.99).

How to Choose Which Bottles are for You

You need to make one crucial choice. Either you 'buy in' to Avent, accepting that their sizing is different to others, and buy the whole system (bottles, brush, teats, steriliser), or you don't. If you know you are going to go the Avent route there are good-value starter packs on sale from virtually every nursery goods supplier. Some include the steriliser but others don't.

The Avent bottles are excellent. However, there are three main reasons to consider standard bottles:

- There is a wide variety of different-shaped teats available for standard bottles.
- If your baby is one of the few who doesn't get on with the Avent silicone teats, you will have to buy a new set of bottles.
- You can probably fit more standard bottles in your steriliser in one go.

Teat Checklist
The Essentials

- You need teats that fit your bottles and teats that are the right 'flow' for your baby (see below).
- You also need more teats than bottles (they tend to disappear or disintegrate during the 3am feed).
- They should meet BS 7368.

Teat Shapes

- Unless you are buying a bottle-feeding starter pack, you will have to buy teats separately. Different babies like different teats, so if your baby seems unhappy (i.e. he dribbles out the feed or seems frustrated by the feeding experience), try a different material or a different-shaped teat.

Orthodontic Teats
- Compared to a normal teat, these have a bulbous, slightly wonky appearance. They are shaped to follow the contours of a baby's mouth. These often work well for babies who are switching from the breast to the bottle.
- The NUK Orthodontic teat (size 1 for babies up to six months) is worth a try if you are not having any success with more easily available models. You can telephone them for stockists on 01438 351341.

Ribbed Teats
- These are teats made for the Pur range by Tommee Tippee. They have external ribbing intended to mimic the maternal nipple.

Wide-Neck Teats
- These only fit wide-neck bottles.

Teat Features
Materials
- Teats are made of either silicone or latex. Silicone is transparent so it is easy to see if it is clean. It is hard-wearing. Latex is softer and less durable.
- Avent bottles only use silicone teats.

Anti-Colic Valves
- These are dents or holes which aim to reduce the amount of air your baby takes in with his milk. (Although not proven, many people believe that too much air causes colic. For advice on colic consult a medical professional.)

Flow
- Teats have different-sized holes to match your baby's sucking ability. So a newborn baby needs a slow flow but an older, hungrier baby can deal with a faster flow.
- If in doubt, look out for a variable-flow teat which releases liquid in proportion to the baby's suck. You will know if the flow is too fast as the baby will seem to be constantly choking and spluttering.

Self-Sealing Caps
- With some bottles, you have to store the teat facing down into the milk with a disc on top to stop leaks. If you are out and about, the extra fiddling could prove an absolute pain.
- The alternative is a self-sealing cap. This is a bottle lid that fits so tightly that you do not need to do this.

Product Table

Standard Feeding Bottles

Brand	Teat	Price	Stockists	Comments
Tommee Tippee	Comes with latex medium-flow teat so you will need to buy a slow-flow teat for a newborn. Latex or silicone.	£1.69 for 125ml £1.79 for 250ml	Independent stores or Tel: 0500 979899	The neck is slightly wider than the average standard bottle, so these are the easiest to fill of those tested. Quantity markings on bottle are not that easy to read. But a good-value, leak-free bottle.
Mothercare Feeding Bottle	Silicone slow-flow fine for a newborn.	£1.30 for 250ml	Tel: 01923 210210	
Boots ☺	Latex medium-flow, so you will need to buy a slow-flow teat for a newborn.	£1.19 for 125ml £1.30 for 250ml	Boots	We love these. They are easy for a baby to grip and the markings stay clear after countless washes. And they are amongst the cheapest around.

Standard Feeding Bottles (continued)

Brand	Teat	Price	Stockists	Comments
Pur Natur Feeder Bottle	Silicone slow-flow, anti-colic valve.	£1.99 for 250ml		Easy to clean; sealing disc has handle for easy removal.
Maws Feeding Bottle	Latex medium-flow.	£1.45 for 125ml £1.55 for 250ml	Tel: 0500 979899	Clear markings, but not so easy to fill.
Cannon Babysafe Standard	Silicone slow-flow.	£1.65 for 125ml £1.79 for 250ml	Tel: 0800 289064	

Wide-Neck Feeding Bottles

Brand	Teat	Price	Stockists	Comments
Avent Feeding Bottle ☺	Silicone slow-flow to reduce colic.	£2.99 for 125ml £3.29 for 250ml	Tel: 0800 289064	Most parents' all-time favourite. Designed by a parent who had suffered with other bottles, this has clear markings, is easy to fill, and easy to travel with, as the cap self-seals.
Tommee Tippee Wide Neck	Silicone slow-flow.	£2.59 for 125ml £2.99 for 250ml	Tel: 0500 979899	Easy-to-read markings, bright and colourful.
Boots Wide Neck	Silicone medium-flow.	£2.09 for 125ml £2.49 for 250ml	Boots	Easy to assemble, clear markings.

Wide-Neck Feeding Bottles (continued)

Brand	Teat	Price	Stockists	Comments
Pur Natur Wide Neck	Silicone slow-flow, anti-colic valve.	£2.55 for 125ml £2.99 for 250ml	Tel: 0500 979899	
Maws Feeding Bottle	Silicone medium-flow.	£2.89 for 250ml	Tel: 0500 979899	

Disposable Bottle Systems

Brand	Teat	Price	Comments
Avent	Special silicone disposable system teats come in two flow rates (£2.29 for two).	Reusable rigid plastic holder and teat sold with 10 pre-sterilised plastic bags and one teat (£3.99) 40 disposable bags (£2.49)	If you have an Avent breast pump you can fit the bags onto the pump and then store breast milk in the freezer for later feeds. You have to buy the disposable teats; you can't use normal Avent ones.
Pur Natur	Three flow rates (£1.99 for two).	As above	Teats will not suit all babies.

Sterilisers

Although bottles need to be scrupulously clean and germ-free, you do not need to buy a steriliser. You can boil bottles, teats and most breast pump accessories in a lidded saucepan for 10 minutes. But, for peace of mind, speed and convenience, most parents opt for a purpose-built sterilising unit. You will need to wash bottles and teats with a bottle brush prior to sterilising them.

You will not need a steriliser once your child is weaned. If you still want to give your bottles a thorough wash, domestic dish-washing machines reach a high temperature that kills most bugs.

Shopping List
- Chemical steriliser *or*
- Microwave steriliser *or*
- Steam steriliser.

Checklist
Brand
- Choose your bottles at the same time as you choose your steriliser, as some have bottles included in the price and you don't want to buy more bottles than you need.
- Also the steriliser must be compatible with your brand of bottles, otherwise you may not be able to fit all your bottles into it.

Capacity
- Ideally, you want to make up one day's bottles first thing in the morning, put them in the fridge and take them out as you need them. In order to do this you need a steriliser that takes six bottles.

Size
- Do you have the space to use and store your preferred type of steriliser?
- Large steam sterilisers and cold water sterilisers will monopolise a small chunk of kitchen worktop while they are in use.

Chemical Sterilisers
- A chemical steriliser is a lidded container that you fill with water, to which you add a sterilising tablet. Bottles soak for around 30 minutes. Bottles then need to be rinsed in boiled water prior to use, as residue may cause an allergic reaction in some babies.
- This is the most fiddly system but if you are mainly breastfeeding this may suit you fine.
- These are good for travelling: all you need is access to clean water for sterilising and newly boiled water for rinsing the bottles afterwards.

Steam Sterilisers
- With a steam steriliser, water is poured into a mains-powered container. Switch on and 10 minutes later you have clean, odour-free bottles.
- If you want speed, convenience, no residues and have the space, go for a steam steriliser. This is a good item to buy second-hand (see pp. 8–12).

Microwave Sterilisers
- Check that the dimensions and wattage of your microwave oven are compatible with the specifications of the steriliser before you buy it. A steriliser can melt if the incorrect wattage is used.
- Not all microwave sterilisers fit inside all microwave ovens.
- Smaller sterilisers have a limited capacity but this may be advantageous when travelling.
- If you are happy with a system that only does four bottles, microwave sterilisers are excellent value.

STERILISERS

Tongs
- Some models come with tongs that you sterilise with your bottles. These allow you to insert teats into their rings without touching them with your hands.

Value
- Microwave sterilisers are the best value but can only do four bottles in one go.
- Also the models available may not fit your microwave oven.

Product Table

Sterilisers		
Model	**Includes**	**Comments**
Cold Water Sterilisers		
Boots Complete Baby Feed Time Steriliser (£17.99) £	Six Boots 250ml feeding bottles with newborn silicone teats Four-week supply of sterilising tablets Bottle brush	A real bargain. The bottles alone would normally cost about £8.40.
Mothercare Six Bottle Cold Water Steriliser (£17.99)	Six 250ml feeding bottles with latex teats Eight sterilising tablets Bottle brush	This is ideal for breastfeeders who just want to sterilise the odd few bits, as there is a lower filling level to allow you to do smaller, more economical batches of sterilising.
Mothercare Four Bottle Cold Water Steriliser (£13.99)	Four 250ml feeding bottles with latex teats Eight sterilising tablets Bottle brush	As above, but smaller.

Sterilisers (continued)

Model	Includes	Comments
Mothercare Disposable Cold Water Steriliser Bags (£6.99)	Seven drawstring bags Seven sterilising tablets	This is expensive, but may suit some travellers. Each bag takes a bottle and its accessories. Hang it on a tap or hook while it's in use. Travellers may find it cheaper and easier in the long term to use a disposable bottle system.
Tommee Tippee Disposable Sterilising Bags (£5.25)	Three drawstring bags Two sterilising tablets	As above.

Steam Sterilisers

Model	Includes	Comments
Avent Steam Steriliser (£35) ☺	Two 250ml feeding bottles with newborn silicone teats Tongs	Takes six wide-neck bottles. Ready in nine minutes.
Babytec Six-Bottle Steriliser (£24.95) £		Can sterilise six bottles of any shape in eight minutes. Its triangular shape means that you can push it into a corner when not in use. Good value.
Babytec Compact Steam Steriliser (£19.95)		Nifty two-bottle steriliser that folds down when not in use.
Boots Feed Time Steam Steriliser (£33)		Will sterilise up to six bottles of any shape in nine minutes.
Lindam Universal Steam Steriliser (£24.99)	Tongs	Will sterilise up to 10 standard or five wide-neck bottles in 12 minutes.
Mothercare Electric Steam Steriliser (£24.99)	Tongs	Rack system for stacking. Holds four bottles (not included). The larger model (£29.99) holds six bottles (not included).

Sterilisers (continued)

Model	Includes	Comments
Microwave Sterilisers		
Avent Microwave Steriliser (£12.99 without bottles; £16.99 with two bottles) ☺	Tongs	Suitable for ovens between 500 and 875 watts. Can do four bottles in eight minutes plus two minutes cooling time.
Boots Microwave Feeding Bottle Steam Steriliser (£15.99)	Four standard bottles	Suitable for ovens up to 1100 watts. Good value if you want to buy bottles as well.
Lindam Microwave Steriliser (£9.99)		Suitable for ovens up to 850 watts. Can do four bottles in eight minutes.
Maws Steriliser Starter Kit (£17.99) £	Four bottles with teats Tongs Bottle brush Eight sterilising tablets	Suitable for all wattages; can also be used as a cold water steriliser. The best value and the most versatile. Especially good when travelling.
Mothercare Four Bottle Microwave Steriliser (£9.99)		Holds four standard or wide-neck bottles. Has a rack system for stacking. Stays sterile for up to three hours.

Bottle-Feeding Accessories

A hundred years ago, babies became ill and many died due to bugs picked up through a feeding bottle. Unlike the purpose-built models of today, this was an old beer bottle with a piece of muslin wedged in the neck for the baby to suck on. Not only has bottle design moved on dramatically since then but there is now a host of associated products available to ensure that your bottles remain clean and germ-free.

Shopping List
- Bottle brushes.
- Bottle carrier.
- Bottle warmer.

Checklist
Bottle and Teat Brushes
- Use these (available from most chemists and some kitchenware shops) to remove all traces of formula before sterilising your bottles.

Bottle Carriers
- These are insulated bags designed to keep milk cool so bacteria cannot breed.
- *Never* put a bottle of warm milk inside as this could encourage the growth of bacteria and make your baby sick.
- You do not need one of these if you have a changing bag because it should contain its own bottle compartment. But if you find a large changing bag unwieldy, these are a good alternative.

Bottle-Feeding Accessories

Bottle Warmers
- These are worth buying if you want to warm a bottle without getting out of bed or out of the car. Some models can be used to heat baby food as well.
- Mine could have been a piece of kitchen sculpture with a little sign saying 'do not touch'. I never got round to using it. But others swear by them – especially for night feeds.
- Your health visitor will strongly advise you against using a microwave oven to heat bottles. Many people ignore this. The real danger with microwaved milk is that it can heat unevenly so that there are 'hot spots' in the milk.
- After heating, leave the bottle for a few minutes and shake it a little (if you dare) to allow the heat to spread evenly. When you think the temperature is about right, let a little milk drip onto the back of your hand just to check.

Bottle Feeding on the Move
It is dangerous to keep a bottle lukewarm for long, as bacteria can grow in the milk. When you are out, it is easier and quicker to heat up a bottle from room temperature than one that is cold from being in the fridge.

There are two safe options:

- If you need at least four feeds, boil the water in advance and put it into the bottles without any formula. Measure out the correct quantities of formula and keep them in a separate storage container ready to mix as required. The Avent Milk Powder Dispenser is a container specially designed to carry measured feeds (£3.99 from most nursery retailers).
- If you only need one feed, the brilliant Umix Shake-It-Up Bottle (£4.99 from Tesco Direct, Tel: 0345 024024) keeps the formula in a compartment in the bottle itself. You twist it round and the formula falls into the water ready for mixing.

Product Table

Bottle and Food Warmers		
Brand and Price	**Stockists**	**Comments**
Avent Bottle and Food Warmer (£19.95)	Tel: 0800 289064	Six minutes to heat 125ml bottle; eight minutes to heat a jar of baby food. Holds all bottles, jars and cans; microwave bowl, light indicator.
Boots Bottle and Baby Food Warmer (£17.99)	Boots	Six minutes to heat 125ml bottle; seven minutes to heat a jar. Holds all bottles, jars and cans; light indicator, cable store for safety.
Babytec Electronic Bottle and Food Heater (£18.95)	Babytec (Tel: 01258 459554)	Three minutes for 125ml bottle; four minutes to heat a jar. Holds all bottles, jars and cans; tripod for jars to alter height for handling.
Lindam Night and Day Feeding System (£29.99)	Tesco Direct (Tel: 0345 024024)	Insulated cooler system with night light. Keeps bottles chilled and warmer section heats bottles in six minutes.
Lindam Universal Bottle Warmer (£14.99)	Tesco Direct (Tel: 0345 024024)	Warms all sizes of bottles and baby food jars. Comes with bowl.
Babytec Car Bottle and Food Heater (£9.95)	Babytec (Tel: 01258 459554) Also Mothercare, and Great Little Trading Company	Plugs into car lighter; takes 15–20 minutes to heat; belt wraps around bottle, jar or can. This one has an integral element so is less fussy than ones that rely on a chemical gel. The latter requires aftercare, but this model does not.

Soothers/Dummies

Soothers are possibly the most emotive item of baby kit. A soother is a teat mounted on a plastic mouthguard that a baby can suck when not eating or drinking. Some have a ring on the front. Do not put this on a ribbon round your baby's neck as this could strangle him. Soothers should meet BS 5239.

The general view seems to be that soothers are fine in the early months but ideally they should be restricted to sleep times, and, after a while, removed altogether. If you remove a soother too soon and your baby is very 'sucky' he may start sucking his thumb, which is far worse, as you cannot restrict use.

Long-term, strong sucking can displace teeth. But the worst dental problems are caused by carers who dip soothers in jam or honey to make them taste good. This can cause serious tooth decay. There can also be potential psychological problems in store for older soother-users. Some practitioners believe that they prevent the development of language and stop a child trying to interact with the outside world.

Be sure to sterilise soothers after use as they can harbour infection.

Checklist
- An orthodontic teat will cause least disturbance to the development of your baby's mouth.
- Buy ones in hard plastic containers that you can wash and keep for storing soothers that are not in use. These are often microwave proof – for easy sterilising.
- Buy two at a time. Soothers are small and get lost easily. If your baby is dependent on a particular make, have a spare to hand in case of emergency.

- Check soothers regularly for tears, as particles may cause your baby to choke.

Preferred soothers are:

- ♛ Mam (from £2.99 for two).
- ☺ Avent (from £2.59 for two).

Breastfeeding Bras

In theory, you don't need to buy anything for breastfeeding. Alison Watts, of the National Childbirth Trust, says, 'It's totally non-consumerist... which doesn't fit well in a consumer society where people view buying things as conferring value to an activity. The gadgets available give the idea that breastfeeding is messy, and possibly expensive.' But of course it isn't – it's free! So, if in doubt give it a try. It's widely recognised as the best start you can give your baby.

If you want help with breastfeeding, the following voluntary organisations have a central telephone number which you can call for details of their local breastfeeding counsellors in your area:

- National Childbirth Trust: 0181 992 8637.
- Association of Breastfeeding Mothers: 0171 813 1481.
- The La Leche League: 0171 242 1278.

Shopping List
- Two to three nursing bras.

Nursing/Feeding Bra Checklist
Type
- As every woman is a different shape, it is impossible to recommend the ultimate bra. We have therefore categorised the types of bra available, so you can test which type suits you.
- If your breasts are very large, go for a front-opening model as you will need maximum support.
- In general, look for a bra that is supportive and easy to open and close; ideally with one hand.

- Comfort is crucial.
- Expect to try on several different models to find a perfect fit.
- Not all women need to buy special nursing bras. You may find your ordinary bras perfectly comfortable while breastfeeding. If so, you can skip this section!

When and Where to Shop
- Buy your first nursing bras towards the end of your pregnancy.
- Six weeks after the birth you will need to go back to the shop for the fitter to check that the bras are supporting you properly.
- Go somewhere where there are trained fitters (e.g. John Lewis or your local NCT supplier).

Support
- The bra should support you at the back as well as the front, without feeling restricted or pinched.
- If it rides up at the back when you move your arms or bend your back forward, it is no good.
- There should be strong support under the breast at the front.

Shape
- It's vital for the bra to cover the whole breast, without skin bulging at the side or over the top. This should help you avoid the problems of blocked milk ducts.
- There should be extra room round your nipples.

Fabric and Construction
- If its edges dig into you, do not buy it.
- The fabric must be breathable (e.g. cotton).
- The straps must be non-elastic, wide and adjustable to ensure a comfortable fit.

Drop-Cup Bras
- These unhook from the shoulder strap.

- They can be flicked open in a second but some have an interior cup that needs to be folded back to fully expose the breast.
- You may find these fiddly to close.

Front-Opening Bras
- More hooks mean better support. This type of bra is usually suggested for women with larger breasts.
- But they can prove tricky to open and close – tiresome if you are planning discreet feeds in public places.

Zip-Cup Bras
- You may have to practise not catching your skin in the bra as you zip these up.
- But they offer immediate exposure and good support.
- Experts can manage to zip and unzip them one-handed.

Sleep Bras and the Alternatives
If you need to wear something at night because you are leaking, you have three choices: sleep on a towel, wear a cropped sports top that will hold breast pads in place (see pp. 59–61), or buy a sleep bra. These do not offer as much support as other types of maternity bras. This is because they must not restrict your breasts in any way.

Buying Bras by Mail Order
If you want to order a bra, you will need someone to help measure your bra size and cup size (see below).

Bra Size
- Wear a bra.
- Ask your fitter to run a tape measure round your ribcage below your breasts (the tape should feel firm but not tight).
- Put your arms by your sides and take a measurement.
- If the measurement is even, add 6 inches. If it is odd, add 5 inches, e.g. 30 + 6 = 36; 33 + 5 = 38.

Cup Size
- Take another measurement round the fullest part of your breasts.
- The difference between this one and the other is your cup size. So if this measurement is 37 and your first measurement was 36: first measurement (fm) + 1 inch = B. You would therefore be a 36B. Cup sizes: fm + 1 inch = B; fm + 2 inches = C; fm + 3 inches = D; fm + 4 inches = DD; fm + 5 inches = E.

Product Table

What we looked for:

- Comfort.
- Ease of use.

Feeding Bras

Brand and Price	Model	Stockists	Comments
Drop-Cup Bras			
Anita (£18.50)	Style 5073 100% cotton	Mothernature (Tel: 0161 485 7359)	Soft but supportive; also ideal during pregnancy. Integrated support panel in cups; seam-free.
Anita (£22)	Kwik Klip Style 5032 65% cotton	Mothernature (as above)	Extra easy to open and close with one hand. Available in black.
Bravado (£22.95)	Maternity Bra 92% cotton	Active Birth Centre (Tel: 0171 561 9006)	Pull-on bra, popper opening on strap, wide back, under-cup elastic. Available in white, black and bold floral print.

Feeding Bras (continued)

Brand and Price	Model	Stockists	Comments
Royce (£19)	Nursing Bra	Tel: 01295 265557	Worth buying if you intend to breastfeed for a while as these wash well.
Emma Jane (£14)	Drop Cup	Tel: 0181 599 3004	Gives good support; comfortable to wear; one-hand release clip.
Front-Opening Bras			
Berlei (£18)	Style 302	John Lewis	Well cut and supportive. A 'cross your heart' design.
Mothercare (£14)	72% cotton	Tel: 01923 240356	Allows easy, discreet breastfeeding.
Zip-Cup Bras			
Emma Jane (£16)	Style 408 45% cotton	Tel: 0181 599 3004	Emma Jane's best-selling bra. Has a protector behind zip.
Boots (£16)	Nursing Bra 39% cotton		White, medium support; wide shoulder straps for comfort and support.
Silhouette (£16.50)	Harmony	John Lewis	
Royce (£16.50)	Nursing Bra	Tel: 01295 265557	

Feeding Bras (continued)

Brand and Price	Model	Stockists	Comments
Mava (£18.75)	Zip Cup	NCT (Mail order: 0141 636 0600)	Particularly good for large cup sizes. 100% cotton lining.
Sleep Bras			
Mothercare (£10)	Sleep Bra		
Mothernature (£10)	Sleep Bra	Mothernature (Tel: 0161 485 7359)	95% cotton; gives light support.
Silhouette (£15.50)	Selina	John Lewis	
Emma Jane (£6.50)	Sleep Bra	Tel: 0181 599 3004	This is more of a crop top.
Mava (£9.75)	Night-time	NCT (Mail order: 0141 636 0600)	Offers light support and lots of lace.

Breastfeeding Accessories

Shopping List
- Breast pads (disposables or reusables).
- Breast shells.
- Nipple cream.
- Nipple shields.
- Breast milk freezer bags/containers.

Checklist
Breast Pads
- Don't buy breast pads until you know whether or not you need to. Most leaking stops by six weeks after the birth.
- Breast pads slip inside your bra and absorb milk that leaks from your nipples. If you find that you are prone to leak whatever you put down your bra, a patterned top will disguise smaller stains.
- You have a choice between disposables (which you buy in packs of 50) or reusables which you can wash in the washing machine. Disposables are more popular but reusables are far better value for long-term use.
- Avoid plastic-backed breast pads, as they can increase the tendency to sore nipples if not changed frequently.
- If you get thrush in the nipple area while breastfeeding throw away your reusable breast pads and buy new ones.
- Available at baby equipment stores and good chemists.

Breast Shells
- Some mothers find that when they are feeding from one side they tend to leak copiously from the other. If this is your experience, you might want to buy breast shells.

- These fit over your nipples and are held in place by your bra to collect milk that can then be stored for a later feed. Only use breast shells for a short period of time and whilst feeding (to avoid problems with blocked milk ducts).
- Available at baby equipment stores and good chemists.

Nipple Creams
- Take advice from your doctor on the best ointment for sore or cracked nipples.
- Available at chemists (e.g. Boots moisturising nipple cream – £1.89).
- Some people reckon that nothing beats a little expressed milk rubbed gently onto the affected area.
- According to the NCT, there's no research evidence for the efficacy of any creams or ointments. Getting your baby on to the breast well and comfortably should help you avoid the problem in the first place.

Nipple Shields
- Experts strongly advise against these, as they reduce milk supply and don't solve the problem of sore, cracked nipples anyway.
- However, they may occasionally be used as a last resort – with help and advice from a midwife.

Product Table

Breastfeeding Accessories		
Type	Brand and Price	Comment
Breast Pads		
Disposable ☺	Johnson & Johnson (30 pads for £2.99)	Very good for heavy leakage – don't slip. Highly recommended.
Disposable £	Boots (50 pads for £2.89)	Good value; absorbency fine for most.

Breastfeeding Accessories (continued)

Type	Brand and Price	Comment
Disposable	Mothercare (40 pads for £2.50)	Good value – fine for most.
Non-disposable	NCT catalogue (four pads for £3.25) Tel: 0141 636 0600	
Non-disposable	Avent (six pads for £4.65)	Good value.
Non-disposable ☺	Kooshies (six pads for £5.95). Available by mail order from Perfectly Happy People (Tel: 0870 6070545)	'Extremely comfortable, breathable and effective,' say long-term breastfeeders. You need two packs.
Breast Shells		
	Avent (two for £4.19)	
	Boots (two for £2.99)	
	Mothercare (two for £4)	
Soothing Breast Packs		
	JoJo Maman Bébé (two for £11.99) Tel: 0171 351 4112	Reusable vinyl breast packs. Can be used warm or cool and fit inside a bra. The alternative to this is a cabbage. Keep it in the fridge and take off the leaves to slip into your bra for cool but faintly odoriferous relief.

Breast Pumps

Expressing by hand is fast, easy, convenient and cost-free (once you've learned the simple technique which your midwife will show you), though many mothers prefer to use a breast pump.

New mothers are not advised to express until their milk production is properly established. This is usually around six weeks after giving birth.

The best type of pump, in terms of effectiveness, is the large electric type. But they are very heavy and cumbersome. One mother told us about a particularly embarrassing incident lugging one of these on the Eurostar which ended up with her having to do a mime to a crowd of disbelieving French customs officials.

Engorged Breasts

If you are having problems with engorged breasts, feed your baby frequently and ring for help from your midwife and/or local voluntary breastfeeding support group.

Checklist

Numerous mothers we interviewed had tried at least two types before settling on a model that worked for them and fitted into their lifestyle.

Manual Pumps
- Although Avent have a model (Isis) that needs less pulling power, you still need good strong hands and wrists or an amazing technique to be successful with a manual pump.
- However, they tend to be cheap and easily portable.

Breast Pumps

Electric Pumps

- ☺ The large, heavy electric pumps, hired from NCT, La Leche or Ameda Egnell, worked exceptionally well for all users.
- But these models are neither discreet nor particularly cheap, costing around £30 per month to hire, plus your own collection kit (£7).

Battery/Mains-Powered Pumps

- Although these did not rate the same 100% satisfaction as the model above (some mothers could not get on with them at all), they were particularly praised by desk-bound working mothers who used these small powered pumps to express in the cloakroom at work.
- 'If you find that you are expressing less and less it may be the batteries running down . . . Get an adaptor (£5.99). It's cheaper in the long run and you'll get consistent results,' advised one mother.

Product Table

What we looked for:

- Effectiveness.
- Ease of use.
- Ease of cleaning.

Breast Pumps

Type	Brand and Price	Stockists	Comments
Manual	Maws (£17.99)	Maws (Tel: 0500 979899), Mothercare	One-handed pump; fits most standard and wide-neck bottles.
Manual	Boots (£15.99)	Boots	One-handed pump; fits most wide-neck bottles; can be tiring on the hands.

Breast Pumps (continued)

Type	Brand and Price	Stockists	Comments
Manual £	Avent Isis (£25)	Avent (Tel: 0800 289064)	Easy finger-grip pump action. Light to carry. Fits Avent disposable bottle bags.
Manual	Ameda Egnell (£14)	Ameda Egnell (Tel: 01823 336362)	One-handed pump; fits most wide-neck bottles; can be tiring on the hands.
Battery or mains (adaptor included) 👑	Mam Medela Mini electric (£49.50)	Mam (Tel: 0121 326 6992)	Generally very popular for comfort and efficiency; fits most standard bottles.
Battery or mains (adaptor included)	Safe and Sound (£29.99)	Safe and Sound (Tel: 01789 299942)	Fits wide-and standard-neck bottles.
Battery or mains (no adaptor included)	Babytec (£21.95)	Babytec (Tel: 01747 823393; Helpline: 01258 459554)	Good value; easy to use.
Mains 👑	Axicare CM5 Electric (£69 plus £3.50 p&p)	Mothernature (Tel: 0161 485 7359)	For home use, as it is heavy; but strong suction and fast results make it a good bet for long-term expressing.

Changing Units and Mats

Some people's backs ache so much after giving birth that a waist-height changing unit is essential. Any solid piece of furniture (chest of drawers, dining room table, cupboard) that reaches your waist and has surface dimensions large enough to accommodate a mat is fine.

However, the safest way to change your baby is by putting him on a changing mat on the floor. Nearly every mother we spoke to on this subject had some horror story about their baby rolling off the bed or changing table. I cannot stress how easy it is for something to happen in that split second when you turn away to dispose of the dirty nappy.

Shopping List
- Changing unit.
- Changing mat.
- Mobile or similar toy to distract baby while changing (see p. 193).

Checklist
Versatility
- Choose a unit that can become a cupboard or chest of drawers once you have finished using it for changing purposes.
- If you are experiencing back problems, a changing table with an integral bath may be of interest.

Stability
- It must have brackets or a means of fixing it against a wall, so larger babies cannot destabilise it.

Safety

- Some changing units have a ridge or high sides round the area where your baby lies. These may stop a baby rolling off, but you should never leave your baby unattended on a changing unit for a second. If you are holding onto your baby the whole time and blocking the longer side with your body, there should be no way that he can roll off.
- Once your baby is bigger, he may find the changing unit very uncomfortable if the high sides are digging into his legs.

Changing Mats

- It seems that the higher the padded sides on these items, the higher the price charged. You do not need high sides, as you should be holding your baby while he is on the mat.
- Don't even think about flannel or fabric changing mats. They may look pretty but if you have to wash them in the machine you will be temporarily matless. Go for good old fully wipeable plastic.

Product Table

Changing Units and Mats

Brand	Model and Price	Stockists	Comments
Changing Units			
Cosatto	Sorrento (£99)	John Lewis, independent retailers	Can use drawers afterwards, though not a thing of beauty. Has rigid bath with drainage pipe.
Monbebe	Monica (£175)	Tel: 01484 401100	Sturdy and versatile. Comes with a bath that becomes a chest of drawers when bath is removed. Has a changing mat top. Fitted with four castors, two of which can be locked.

Changing Units and Mats (continued)

Brand	Model and Price	Stockists	Comments
Mothercare	Dresser with Bath (£139)	Tel: 01923 240365	Pine dresser with integral bath and drainage pipe. Converts into shelving unit. Does not come with changing mat but a standard one fits it.
Cosatto	Roma (£190)	Tel: 01268 452288	Drawer unit with bath. Has padded changing mat and handy shelf for towels and nappies. Converts into chest of drawers.
Monbebe	Esther (£60)	Tel: 01484 401100	Useful unit if you do not have much space, as it folds flat once bath is removed. Has a storage shelf and changing mat.
Bébécar	American Dresser (£115)	John Lewis	In natural wood or white; good quality; has three shelves; packs flat. Height 80cm.
Mamas and Papas	Rosella (£99)	John Lewis	Made of wood and MDF; if you are concerned about baby rolling off, this has an extra-high bar. Height 103cm.
Mamas and Papas ☺	Jackie (£74.95)	Independent retailers	Two PVC shelves; plastic tray for accessories; padded PVC changing mat covering bath; water drainage pipe.
Changing Mats			
Mothercare	Tweet Dreams (£7)	Tel: 01923 240365	Standard size with raised sides. Bright and fun design.
East Coast	Selection (£6.50 to £14.75)	John Lewis	The higher the price, the higher the edges.

Changing Units and Mats (continued)

Brand	Model and Price	Stockists	Comments
Tesco	Fold and Go Changing Kit (£6.99)	Tesco Direct (Tel: 0345 024024)	Has a nappy pocket and folds neatly into own bag for portability.
JoJo mail order ☺	Travel Changing Mat (£7.99)	Tel: 0171 351 4112	Has inflatable sides. Recommended on basis that it is ideal for home use on a changing table but deflates for travelling.

Cots and Cot Beds

'How do you choose the perfect cot?' I asked an assistant in one top store. She replied, 'What I say to my customers is: choose the cot and the mattress you would choose to sleep on yourself.'

Looking round the shop at assorted grandmothers and pregnant women, my mind boggled at the thought of these ladies attempting to squeeze themselves into a Cossato Carolina 'with playball feature'.

I am still none the wiser on how you choose 'the best'. It seems to be down to individual taste and budget.

Shopping List
- Crib and bedding.
- Cot/cot bed.
- Cot mattress.
- Moses basket.
- Nursery thermometer.
- Travel cot.

Checklist
Cots Versus Cot Beds
- On putting up a cot bed: 'It was very awkward for tired Dad to self-assemble ... one of the holes had to be re-bored. What should have been a 30-minute job took three hours. Even worse ... we have decided to put it in the spare room so it has to be completely dismantled and rebuilt.'
- There is little difference in price.

- A cot usually has a drop-side mechanism but a cot bed does not. A drop-side is useful. It allows you to reach the mattress without having to bend over the cot-side to put your sleepy baby down.
- A cot will last your baby until he is two or until he starts climbing out.
- A cot bed is larger, converts into a child's bed and can be used until a child is around six. As these are low, it's less traumatic when a child falls out of one than out of a bed of a normal height.
- Cot beds are preferable if you are expecting more than one baby. You can convert the cots into beds at the pace of each child.
- Cot bed linen can be hard to find and expensive.

Cots Only

- Give the cot a good shake and see if it moves, as it must withstand a bouncing toddler.
- Different models allow you to move the mattress either higher or lower within the frame so you don't have to bend right down to pick your baby up. But don't pay more for multiple levels. In reality you only need two.
- Will the shop come and assemble it for you? This is a job for a DIY expert.
- Some models come with teething rails – clear plastic guards that slide onto the sides. If your child is a 'chewer' these will keep the cot rails pristine.

Cot Beds Only

- If you want it to last, avoid any design that might appear too babyish to a five-year-old football fan.
- Ask if you can see how it looks in both its cot and bed modes. Sometimes the ends look out of proportion in the bed incarnation.

Cribs/Cradles

- These are decorative small cots for infants that allow you to rock your baby to sleep.
- They often come with optional decorative extras such as elaborate drapery.

- You need an MA in DIY to assemble one of these.
- These are not appropriate for babies who can sit up.
- Cribs and cradles must conform to BS EN 1130:1997.

Cots and Safety

Cots must conform to BS EN 716:1996. This encompasses the latest thinking on product safety. There are some other precautions you need to be aware of:

- Ensure that you know how to make up a cot so that your baby is lying in the 'feet to foot' position, with his feet to the foot of the cot so that he can't wriggle down and get his head covered with bedding. Leaving large soft toys in the cot may also cause your baby to get too hot.
- Remove mobiles as soon as your baby can sit up and don't leave any toys in the cot that may encourage a larger baby to vault out of it.
- Never position a cot directly under a window or by a radiator or other source of heat.

Product Table

Cots and Cot Beds			
Brand	**Model and Price**	**Stockists**	**Comments**
Under £100			
Ikea	Gök (£35)		Melamine ends with beech slatted sides.
Mothercare	Salisbury (£60)	Tel: 01923 240365	One drop-side, three-position height base, curved end rails, dowels all round.
Mothercare	Chepstow (£59.99)	Tel: 01923 240365	Solid wood, white finish, three-position height base, drop-side.
Ikea £	Gulliver (£60)		Dowels on four sides, fixed sides, three-position height base.

Cots and Cot Beds (continued)

Brand	Model and Price	Stockists	Comments
Babies 'R' Us	Avignon (£79.99) Also see Toulouse Cot (£20 more but exceptional value)		Slats on four sides, two-position base, drop-side.
Continenta	(£99.99, includes mattress)	Index	Adjustable mattress base, drop-side, slats on all sides, choice of white or natural wood finish.

Under £200

Brand	Model and Price	Stockists	Comments
Continenta	ABC (£140)		Slats all round, two-position height base, one-handed drop-side, teething rail, ABC engraving.
Mamas and Papas Cot Bed £	Carla (£105)		Cot bed with dowel and fixed sides, three-position height base, solid end panels. Converts into junior bed.
Mothercare	Playbeads (£150)	Tel: 01923 240365	Solid beech with playbeads on end panel. Slats all round, two-position height base, one-handed drop-side, teething rail.
Index	Francesca, made by Saplings (£129, includes mattress)		Three-height base, drop-side, slats all round. Quilt and bumper set also included but only appropriate for older babies.

Cots and Cot Beds (continued)

Brand	Model and Price	Stockists	Comments
Over £200			
Continenta Cot Bed	Viola (£250)		Colourful cot bed, dowel and fixed sides, two-position mattress, solid end panels.
Cosatto	Orleans (£290)		Rocking base, drawer, teething rail, slats all round, two-position mattress, one-handed drop-side.
Mothercare	Scroll (£200)		Scrolled legs, solid end panels, slatted sides, two-position mattress, one-handed drop-side, teething rail.
Cosatto Cot Bed	Dauphine (£795)	John Lewis	Very top of the range – converts into a sofa. Beech frame, mahogany finish, one drop-side, one fixed, two castors, teething rail. Height 110cm, length 150cm, width 80cm.

Cradles

Brand and Price	Stockists	Comments
Littlewoods Swinging Cradle (£57)	Littlewoods catalogue (Tel: 0345 888222)	Comes complete with mattress for home assembly. Broderie anglaise polycotton accessories are available (£28).
Brio Swinging Cradle (£59)	John Lewis	Available in white/antique pine with birch frame. Mattress is 38cm × 89cm. Comes flat-packed for self-assembly.

Buying Second-Hand Cots

- A reasonably new cot should comply with BS EN 716:1996. Without this it does not conform to the latest safety standard and could be dangerous.
- If it is dismantled be wary. Cots can be damaged when taken apart.
- It should have instructions on assembly.
- Do not consider a cot without its original screws. Using the wrong ones could cause the whole thing to collapse.
- Look at the wood on both the base and the sides. Reject anything with cracks or splits.
- Do not buy a cot with damaged springs.
- Cots that have been repainted are potentially highly dangerous unless the sellers can prove to you that lead-free, non-toxic paint has been used.
- Ensure the drop-side mechanism runs smoothly.
- See pp. 8–12 for general advice on buying second-hand goods.

Cot Mattresses

Following scares associated with cot death (Sudden Infant Death Syndrome), it is commonly believed that you should never buy mattresses second-hand.

After extensive research, including a comprehensive three-year study by a Department of Health Working Group, no evidence has been found to substantiate the 'toxic gas' theory promoted by the Cook Report early in the 1990s. If you have any worries, you can always call the Foundation for the Study of Infant Deaths (FSID) 24-hour helpline on: 0171 235 1721.

It doesn't matter what kind of mattress you use, as long as:

- It is firm, not soft.
- It doesn't sag.
- It shows no signs of deterioration.

Keep it well-aired and clean. Mattresses with a PVC surface or a removable washable cover are easiest to keep clean. Ventilated mattresses (with holes) are not necessary. FSID say: 'We do get parents calling our helpline confused about how to put their baby in feet to foot position if their heads are supposed to be over the holes. It is OK for the baby's head to be on the plastic area.' Never put your baby to sleep on a pillow, cushion, bean bag, water bed or sofa. Mattresses should conform to BS 1877 part 10: 1997.

Checklist
Fit
- The gap between the mattress and the side of the cot should be no more than 4cm.

Thickness
- Look for a mattress that is 8cm–10cm thick.

Cleaning
- Until your baby is in residence, you won't know whether he is the type to regularly leak and posset on his bedding. But the key rule is to go for a mattress that you can wipe clean in moments, as most mattress maintenance takes place at 3am with a baby screeching on your shoulder.
- You can be extra safe with a waterproof undersheet (see p. 82).

Foam/Ventilated Foam
- These are light, good-value items, which many mothers swear by. They are made solely of foam. The top half often has holes so that dribble and vomit can drain away from your baby's face. The bottom part is covered in PVC or a water-resistant material.
- If a baby constantly dribbles on the foam and this is not acted upon, the mattress may go mouldy and will have to be changed. But these mattresses are easily cleaned. If you buy a two-part model (e.g. the Rochingham Dupla) you can just zip off the top half and hand-wash it. It will air-dry eventually.
- Don't put an entire mattress in the wash as it will stay sodden for weeks.

Spring Interior
- The ultimate in comfort for the older baby, these contain springs wrapped in foam padding. They often have PVC covering one side and fabric on the other.
- Liquid rarely penetrates past the covers, so you can just wash the mattress covers according to the manufacturer's instructions.

Natural Fibres
- These mattresses are made from several different fibres including coir coated in latex, cotton, wool and polyester. The breathable fabric that covers the mattress will provide natural ventilation but also hold fluid on the surface.

- When cleaning these mattresses you must be careful not to rub liquids in. Take the cover off carefully to wash it. If the filling is rubber-coated coir and liquid has penetrated the core, simply put your shower head close to the accident site and run clean water through the mattress until you have dispersed the mess out the other side. This is a very, very rare occurrence. Again, it will take a long time to dry, as you must leave it to dry naturally.

Fire Retardants

Although there is no proven link between cot death and mattresses containing antimony, phosphorus or arsenic, the following brands do not use any of these chemicals in their manufacture:

ABC, Babywise, Bébécar, Continenta, Cosatto, Cotsafe, Cradlesafe, Jigsaw, Natural Furniture Co., Reylon, Rochingham (makers of Visivent), Rockliffe, Wilkes.

Mothercare (own brand) and Mamas and Papas contain no added antimony or arsenic but they do contain a non-hazardous phosphorus retardant.

Allergic Babies

If there are allergies in the family that your baby is likely to inherit, take advice on bedding from your hospital paediatrician when he/she comes to check on your baby after the birth. Ask if he/she thinks you need a particular sort of mattress or mattress cover. You may wish to have *The Healthy House* mail order catalogue to hand as this contains anti-allergy bedding cases and dust-mite-proofed goods amongst its products (Tel: 01453 752216).

Product Table

Cot Mattresses			
Brand	**Range**	**Price**	**Stockists**
ABC	Foam and fibre	From £25	Independent retailers
Argos	Foam	From £14.99	Tel: 0870 600 1010

Cot Mattresses (continued)

Brand	Range	Price	Stockists
Mothercare	Full range of mattresses	From £29.99	Tel: 01923 240365
Rochingham (Makers of Golden Slumber, Saferest, Kumfy Sprung and Visivent ranges)	Full range of mattresses	From £25	All large baby product retail outlets. (Rochingham have recently pioneered a new mattress cover that stops liquid permeating the coir but still allows the mattress to breathe.)
Wilkes	Hand-made, natural fibre mattresses, made to order if necessary	From £70	Tel: 01432 268018

Many cot manufacturers, such as Bébécar, Continenta, and Mamas and Papas, will supply own-brand mattresses to go with their cots.

Baby Bedding

Many baby catalogues feature tempting displays of co-ordinating nursery linens. However, the Foundation for the Study of Infant Death (FSID), the UK's leading cot death charity, advises against quilts, duvets and pillows for babies under one.

If your baby is under a year old, use one or more layers of light blankets. Don't swaddle or use sheepskins, electric blankets or hot water bottles.

Acrylic cellular blankets are popular in colder homes, as they are soft, washable and warm; 100% wool does not wash well in some machines – a major drawback.

Baby sleeping bags are increasingly popular as, unlike sheets, they cannot be kicked off on a cold night. If your baby is a restless sleeper and he tends to wake when he is uncovered, these could be for you. FSID recommends that these sleeping bags be:

- Low tog (no more than 1.5).
- Sleeveless and hoodless.
- Well-fitting – not too big or too small.
- Designed so that you can easily feel your baby's tummy to check whether he is too hot.

> Remember – if your baby sleeps in a sleeping bag he may not need any bedclothes.

Specialist baby sleeping bag mail order firm Kiddycare offer an extensive selection. Telephone for a brochure: 01309 674646.

Shopping List
- Four cotton cellular blankets.

- Four top sheets.
- Four bottom (fitted) sheets.
- Mattress protector.
- Room thermometer.

Things *Not* to Buy

Product	Reasons
Pillow	Babies need to lose heat out of the tops of their heads; pillows can lead to a baby getting too hot.
Cot bumper	If a baby sleeps with his head rammed against one of these, it can hamper natural heat loss. Once he is sitting up, he may try to use these to lever himself out of the cot.
Shawls/receiving blankets	You may want to carry your baby in a blanket but do not swaddle him.
Wedges	To reduce the risk of cot death, you should sleep your baby on his back. FSID advises against the use of wedges which encourage side sleeping unless you have received strong medical advice to do so.

Room Thermometers

Understandably, a lot of parents worry about their babies becoming over-heated. Many retailers will sell you a room thermometer.

If your baby is wearing a nappy, vest and sleepsuit and is covered by a sheet, you can use the thermometer in conjunction with your blankets as follows:

22–24°C	sheet only
20–22°C	one blanket
18–20°C	two blankets
16–18°C	three blankets
12–14°C	four or more blankets

Room thermometers should not be relied on exclusively. One highly experienced retailer told me that the system outlined above really worried her because it takes common sense out of childcare.

Not all babies have the same sensitivity to temperature and it is better to concentrate on how your baby looks and feels rather than just what the thermometer says.

If your baby is sweating or his tummy feels hot to the touch, take off some bedding. Don't worry if your baby's hands or feet feel cool – this is normal.

Checklist
Fitted Bottom Sheets
- These are essential, as they stay smooth and comfortable throughout the night.
- If you are cutting down old sheets for your cot, JoJo (Tel: 0171 351 4112) can supply cot sheet fasteners (£3.99 plus p&p for a packet of four). These are clips on strong elastic that go under the mattress to hold a flat sheet as taut as a fitted one.

Cotton Interlock Sheets
- These soft cotton jersey sheets are ideal for year-round use. They're usually made into fitted sheets to cover the mattress.

Flannelette Sheets
- These are usually made of woven cotton with a brushed cotton texture.

Terry/Stretch Terry Sheets
- Fine towelling – usually cotton mix unless stated.

Stockists
- Stockists include all major nursery retailers and catalogues selling nursery goods. Prices start at around £12 for a packet of four fitted terry sheets (Index).
- Cot bed sheets are hard to find and tend to be pricey but the Tesco *Baby and Toddler Catalogue* (Tel: 0345 024024) sell a variety at around £9.99 for two.
- For something 'special', such as cellular blankets with a crochet trim, ring Clair de Lune for their catalogue

(Tel: 0161 283 4476/7). Prices vary from shop to shop. They will send you a list of retailers in your area.
- Choice mail order catalogue – *Mums & Little Ones* – have a good-value selection, e.g. £24.99 for four white flannelette sheets and a cotton blanket (Tel: 0645 100200).

Product Table

Mattress Protectors

Brand	Model and Price	Stockists	Comments
Great Little Trading Company ♛	Wet-N-Dry (£19.99)	Tel: 0990 673008	Models with a high plastic/PVC content can be very hot for a baby to lie on. This one is made of treated cotton and does the job with 'no sweat'. It can also be used on single beds so it will last longer than other models.
Boots	Protective Cot Sheet (£6)	Boots stores (and home delivery, Tel: 0845 840 1000)	100% PVC. Machine-washable.
Jonelle	Waterproof Glove Sheet (£5)	John Lewis	Waterproof fitted sheet with cellular panels.
Mothercare	Mattress and Sheet Protector (£14.99)		Quilted surface with waterproof backing; machine-washable. Can also be used on single beds.

Moses Baskets

Your baby may well grow out of a Moses basket in a matter of weeks which is why, in retrospect, a number of mothers felt that these were a complete waste of money. When you take your baby outdoors, you will have to transfer him into a pram or car seat, as the Moses basket is really only appropriate for use around the home.

Shopping List
- Wicker Moses basket *or*
- Palm Moses basket.
- Stand (if you want your baby to sleep in basket at night).

Checklist
- A Moses basket should conform to BS 6595: 1985 (baby nests).
- A Moses basket is worthwhile if you need a light portable bed for the early days. Parents of multiples may find them useful.
- But remember that you should not carry your baby around in the basket. Unlike a car seat there are no restraints and no protection; one trip on the stairs and your baby could be catapulted into the wall.
- Do not be swayed by the bedding. Moses baskets are sold 'dressed' with frilly skirts and a matching quilt. The Foundation for the Study of Infant Death suggests that sheets and blankets should be used rather than the quilt.

Wicker Moses Baskets
- This is the 'heirloom' version that will withstand generations of small babies. These baskets are relatively heavy and tend to be larger (*not* recommended for mothers with bad backs).

Palm Moses Baskets
- These are cheaper and lighter but handles may fray over time.

Moses Basket Stands
- You will be encouraged to buy one of these. They are usually sold as an 'extra' which adds around £13.99 (from Index) to the price of the basket. The reasons for buying one of these are that sleeping on the floor may make your baby susceptible to draughts or the unwelcome attentions of pets and siblings.

Alternatives to a Moses Basket

These include the carrycot option on your buggy, a fully reclining baby chair for the odd snooze during the day, or a travel cot. A cot with an easily removable side that you can put next to your own bed can be seen at large branches of Mothercare (ask for the Bedside Cot by Brio, £199). A new baby can also sleep in a proper cot but you will need to fold the sheets low down on the mattress and create an extra-short bed so that your baby cannot get tangled in a vast expanse of bedding. Your community midwife will show you how.

Product Table

Moses Baskets			
Brand	Model	Price	Stockists
Clair de Lune £	Full range, including Austrian broderie anglaise; palm	£28 (wooden stand £18)	Index and independent retailers (Tel: 0161 283 4476/7 or E-mail: sales@Clair-de-lune.co.uk, for brochure)
Mamas and Papas	Classica, palm	£70	Through Mamas and Papas stockists

Moses Baskets (continued)

Brand	Model	Price	Stockists
Zorbit	Noah's Ark/My Garden Design	£49.99 (wooden stand £14.99)	John Lewis and independent retailers
Simon Cameron	Hand-made wicker baskets		Tel: 01531 635046
Continenta	Broderie anglaise	£65	Independent retailers (Tel: 0181 519 9191 for brochure and details of local stockists)

Medicine Cabinet

As far as a toddler is concerned, the healing powers of plasters are magical – but only if they have Winnie-the-Pooh on them. The bog-standard beige doesn't seem to have any effect at all. It therefore makes sense to be prepared for the bumps and bruises that inevitably accompany your baby's physiological achievements – whether this is the pain of cutting a tooth or a crash on the floor as he starts learning to walk.

It is very difficult to gauge the severity of a baby's discomfort. But *if you are worried, contact your GP or the hospital unit where you had your baby.*

Consult a doctor immediately if your baby:

- Has a fever that does not respond to infant paracetamol.
- Has an unusually intense pain that is not colic.
- Has a fit or loses consciousness.
- Has severe watery, smelly diarrhoea and/or repeated vomiting.
- Refuses more than one feed.

Even for minor problems, items in an adult's first-aid kit may not be appropriate for a baby or toddler. For instance, you can't explain to a baby that it isn't a good idea to bite a thermometer and swallow the mercury. Similarly, the dosage in adult medicines may be inappropriate for children.

You therefore have two choices. You can either buy a 'ready-made' model (such as ABC's Child First Aid Kit for £24.99 from independent retailers, or the Great Little Trading Company's Childminder First Aid Kit for £31.99) and add everyday items such as junior paracetamol. Or you can make up a kit yourself.

If you need to keep medicines in a child's bedroom, the Great Little Trading Company Child Safe (£17.99) is a cabinet that can only be opened by adult fingers.

Product Table

Medicine Cabinet	
Product	**What to Buy**
Antiseptic spray	Savlon child's spray does not sting as much as the adult alternative.
Bandages (and strong stainless steel scissors and safety pins)	Have a selection of bandages for emergencies, such as eye pads, sterile bandages, triangular bandage, at least four gauze swabs, wound dressings.
Calamine lotion	Good for rashes.
Decongestants	You can either go the inhalant route with Karvol capsules (10 for £1.79) or suck out secretions with a nasal decongestor (£1.50). (First Years) Nuk nasal decongestor (£2.85).
Infant paracetamol (For babies over three months)	Sugar-free Calpol Infant Suspension (£2.99 for 140ml) or Disprol Infant Sugar-free Paracetamol Suspension (£2.15 for 200ml).
Medicine dropper	Ensures that you give the correct dosage without spilling. Boots (£1.49).
Nail cutters/scissors	You have a choice between nail scissors with rounded tips or baby nail clippers. Both cost around £1.50 from chemists.
Nappy rash cream	Choose between Sudocrem (£2.29 for 125g), Drapolene, or zinc and castor oil cream. Or try painting the rash with egg white or simply leaving the rash exposed to the air.
Plasters	Children's plasters with designs (e.g. Boots Winnie-the-Pooh Child plasters for £1.99) are available at supermarkets and chemists.
Skin cream	E45 cream or oily cream from pharmacy counters.
Sterile dressings, micropore tape	Micropore tape is hypoallergenic and will hold dressings in place.
Teething gel (For babies over four months)	Choose between Bonjela (£2.39), Rinstead (£1.85) or homeopathic alternatives, all at Boots (see section p. 250).

Medicine Cabinet (continued)	
Product	**What to Buy**
Thermometer ♛	Braun Thermoscan is madly expensive (at £39.99) but superb. Incredibly accurate; takes temperature in seconds via insertion in ear. Digital thermometers are battery-driven and cost around £7.99 at all chemists. Forehead thermometers (e.g. Boots Feverscan for £2.70) give a reading in seconds but are not as precise as the others. They are great value and worth knowing about if your baby objects to the other types.
Tweezers	

Homeopathic Remedies

A box of homeopathic remedies by Weleda, covering common first-aid problems, is available for £32.20 plus p&p from NCT Sales (Tel: 0141 636 0600).

Monitors

Baby monitors should not be used as a substitute for checking your baby in person. A monitor allows you to listen to your baby in the nursery while you are elsewhere in the house or garden. It has two units: one that you keep with you to listen in; the other that stays near the baby. This picks up and transmits the sounds he makes.

You do *not* need a monitor if your baby is always in the room with you, or you can hear your baby cry throughout your home.

Shopping List
- Plug-in monitor *or*
- Portable monitor *or*
- Rechargeable monitor *or*
- Video monitor.

Checklist
- Because monitors rely on radio waves, certain environments create too much disturbance for reliable use (keep your receipt handy in case this applies to you).
- And if you are only going to use batteries and never the mains prepare yourself for a major expense.

Plug-in Monitors
- Baby unit plugs into 13 amp socket within three metres of baby; parental unit plugs into a 13 amp socket near the listener.
- Best for carers who will remain in one room while listening to their baby.

Portable Monitors
- Both units work on either mains electricity via an adaptor or batteries. Adaptors are included in price but batteries are not. In theory, the parents' unit picks up sound from 100 metres away.
- Best for carers who want to wander around with listening device.

Rechargeable Monitors
- As above, but parents' unit contains a sealed rechargeable battery that lasts up to three years. These are therefore the most cost-effective option for people wanting heavy-duty usage.
- Best for carers as above, who intend to use the monitor for many hours at a time and who are expecting to keep it in use for a following baby.

Video Monitors
- These allow you to see and hear your baby on a television screen.
- They are ten times the price and more likely to be of use to monitor mischievous toddlers (or a suspect nanny).

Special Features
- Some monitors have a built-in night light. This should give your baby's room a soft glow and you should not have to buy an additional nightlight. However, as plugs are often sited low on the wall, you may find it lights up little more than a few legs of furniture.
- A receiving light on the parents' monitor confirms that all is operating correctly.

Two Channels
- If there are other babies in the neighbourhood, it is essential to buy a monitor with a choice of channels, otherwise you may end up picking up the same frequency on a different monitor in a neighbouring household and you will be listening in on the wrong child.

- If you have bought a Tomy monitor and you are experiencing these sorts of problems it really is worth ringing the Tomy Careline (01703 662600) as they have a good after-sales policy on this.

Visual Indicator/Sound and Light Display
- This allows you to turn off the sound and tell by glancing at a panel of lights whether your baby is crying. The more lights that are flashing, the louder the screams. If you are going to be listening in a room where other people will resent hearing a baby crying, these are a good idea.

Low-Volume Safety Feature
- On models with adjustable volume on the parents' unit, this is a pre-set minimum volume to ensure that you do not turn the monitor so low that you cannot hear your baby.

Product Table

What we looked for:

- Value for money.
- Clear reception.
- Stand-up/clip-on features.

All the audio monitors mentioned here can be mains-operated and transmit by radio waves.

Nursery Monitors			
Model	Brand and Price	Stockists	Comments
Monitors (Aural)			
Plug-in £	Lindam: Baby Talk (£14.99)	Mothercare and independent retailers	Basic model; lacks useful features of Tomy plug-in

Nursery Monitors (continued)

Model	Brand and Price	Stockists	Comments
Plug-in	Boots Plug-In Baby Listener (£21.99)	Boots	Basic model, on the expensive side. Includes night light.
Plug-in £	Tomy: Baby Link (£17.99)	Children's World, independent retailers and Index	'Power on' indicators, two channels, adjustable volume on parents' unit.
Portable	Boots Portable Baby Listener (£27.99)	Boots	Good value, includes light display, a transmission range of 100m, light to indicate sound levels, two channels, low-volume safety feature.
Portable £	Tomy: Walkabout 2000 (£28.50 – varies)	Most baby equipment retailers	Hugely popular model with all features of Boots model and an out-of-range indicator and belt clip.
Portable	Johnson & Johnson Baby Reassurance Monitor (£89)	Boots and independent retailers	Measures baby's sound, room temperature and breathing via a sensor pad on the mattress. Not for the faint-hearted. The baby breathing patterns may freak you out: they can be irregular. If you're not medically trained, it's hard to know what is 'normal'.
Recharge-able	Boots Recharge-able Baby Listener (£35.99)	Boots	Identical features to Boots portable listener with extra facility to recharge the parents' unit.

Nursery Monitors (continued)

Model	Brand and Price	Stockists	Comments
Rechargeable ☺	Tomy: Recharge-About (£39.99)	Baby equipment retailers	Similar to Tomy Walkabout 2000 on p. 93 but has a rechargeable battery. If used for many years the additional expense may be justified.
Rechargeable	Safe and Sound Super Compact Rechargeable (£34.99)	John Lewis and independent retailers	This is the 'bargain' model but it lacks a visual display and the antenna might dig into you if you want to wander around with it clipped on your belt.
Monitors (Visual/Apnoea)			
Aural/visual	Lindam Baby Talk Sound and Vision £330	Great Little Trading Company, Mothercare and Tesco Direct	Uses infra-red technology and has its own screen.
Breathing/ Apnoea	Axminster £250–£350 or hire	Axminster Electronics (Tel: 01297 32360)	Usually only recommended when there is a strong possibility of Sudden Infant Death Syndrome (SIDS). For this monitor to have any purpose, the carer in charge must know how to resuscitate a baby. But even then, you cannot be sure that you will be able to prevent the baby's death.

Nappies

Even the colour of a baby's faeces is deemed suitable dinner party conversation by some besotted parents – maybe they read the same article as I did on how the word 'nappy' is derived from 'napkin'. Before this information is taken to its logical conclusion (darlings, we've run out of serviettes, so I thought we could use . . .) I will move on.

A good nappy is not hard to find. As we speak, scientists all over the developed world are racing to expand nappy technology in a bid to colonise as many bottoms as possible. For nappies are big business. In his first year a baby will use around 2000 nappies. This costs around £900 for disposables or £350 for reusables plus washing bills.

Shopping List
- Nappies in the correct size for your baby (disposable or reusable).
- Night-time nappies.
- Nappy sacks.
- Lidded rubbish bin/Sangenic.

The Ecological Pros and Cons
There are ecological arguments as to whether parents should use disposables or reusables. Each side has come up with their own reasons as to why theirs are the best but the Consumer Association's *Which?* report says: 'Environmentally, there is no clear leader. Certainly, disposables produce far more waste than washable ones but studies into which option uses more energy, raw materials and water overall . . . have arrived at contradictory conclusions.'

The *Which?* study concluded that, for most British people, the most ecologically sound way to protect your baby's bottom was to use reusable nappies that were washed by a nappy service.

Disposable Nappies

Checklist
- For your baby's early days, cheaper brands are fine as he won't be making huge deposits for a while.
- Once he is older, premium nappies do seem worth the extra money as they are more absorbent. Fewer leaks = less washing.
- Always buy the right size. If you get them too big, they will leak.
- If you find your baby needs a more absorbent nappy at night, try night-time nappies (readily available).
- Don't always buy in bulk. Your baby will grow so quickly that you may suddenly find yourself with a stack of nappies that are too small.
- Nappies can be delivered to your door by high street retailers – see Product Table overleaf.
- Be careful not to put nappy-creamed fingers near the nappy fastenings as it stops them sticking. If you tend to do this, keep a roll of Sellotape handy – otherwise you'll waste the nappy.

Half-Price Pampers
If you don't mind buying a month's supply of nappies at once, you can get them from Huntleigh Hygiene (Tel: 01756 706010). As they usually supply nappies to nursing homes, their minimum order is one case (six large packs). They only stock certain Pampers sizes but if they have what you want, they deliver to your door within four working days. The nappies will cost around half what you would pay in a retail outlet.

Disposing of Disposables

Before throwing your nappies away, you can put them in nappy sacks, small, deodorised plastic bags (£1.79 for 75 at all nursery stores). If you can't be bothered – any well-sealed plastic bag will do.

A Sangenic (£21.99 at all nursery stores) is a bin specially designed for nappies. Each time you put a nappy in the Sangenic it is wrapped in deodorised plastic. After two days, you have a string of plastic-coated nappies that you throw away. You need to buy additional cartridges (£2.99 each) containing the plastic wrapping for a month's worth of nappies. If you can't stand the smell of nappy deodoriser this is not for you.

Product Table

Prices fluctuate considerably. Costs shown are for rough guidance and reflect the average cost of a newborn-size nappy.

Disposable Nappies		
Brand	**Home Delivery**	**Comments**
Pampers Baby Dry Extra and Pampers Premiums which have strips of baby lotion to keep skin soft ♕	Boots (Tel: 0845 840 1000), Index (in 48 hours, Tel: 0800 349939), Mothercare (Tel: 01923 240365), Tesco Direct (Tel: 0345 024024 – bargain bulk 'Jumbo' buys available, see catalogue)	Cost: 19p each. Hugely popular, no leaks reported and fastenings work well.
Huggies ♕	Boots (see above), Choice (Tel: 0645 100200), Tesco Direct (see above)	Cost: 18p each. Also have a large following and performed well in testing.

Disposable Nappies (continued)

Brand	Home Delivery	Comments
Sainsbury's Performers £		Cost: 14p each. Testers really liked these. Thought fastenings were particularly good.
Tesco Ultra Dry £	Tesco Direct (see above)	Cost: 14p each. Testers who 'loved' Pampers 'liked' these, as they thought they were similar.
Boots High Performance	Boots (see above)	Cost: 15p each. A good-value nappy for the right-shaped bottom.

Also tested and rated 'OK' were: Superdrug (fine for small babies); Asda nappies (found fastenings not sticky enough); Tickety Boo (liked fastenings but not absorbency).

Reusable Nappies

Some mothers we spoke to liked these, on the grounds that they were easy to use, good value, and perceived as environmentally sound. Others found that their enthusiasm waned once their babies got onto heavy-duty solid foods.

Biodegradable liners mean that you no longer have to scrape waste off nappies and down the toilet prior to washing. You simply flush the liner and contents down the toilet. If you find this a bore, keep a few disposables to hand for easy changing while out and about.

Tracking down the perfect reusable can be tricky. It takes a brave father to go into the local chemist and enquire for Poopers or Bumkins but most brands are available by mail order. The Real Nappy Association can send you information on cloth nappy brands. Send a large SAE to: PO Box 3704, London SE26 4RX.

Checklist
Terry Nappies
- These are traditional nappies that you fold over your baby and fasten with safety pins or Nappy Nippas – plastic grips that are safer and easier to use than a pin (Tel: 01736 351263).
- Terries are cheap and dry quickly.

Shaped Nappies
- These are shaped like a disposable nappy and often have elasticated waists and legs.
- They can take up to eight hours to dry.
- All-in-one shaped nappies have integral waterproofing.
- The two-piece type require additional plastic pants to be worn on top of the nappy. These tend to be far quicker to wash. Poopers, for example, reckon that their polycotton

nappy is virtually dry when it comes out of the washing machine and can be tumble-dried in under five minutes.
- If you are going the 'shaped' route, it is worth buying a trial nappy before you invest in the whole system. If a brand does not suit your baby's contours, you will discover that he is a 'handful' in more ways than one. Most mothers experiment with at least two types before making a full investment.
- When you are trialling your nappies, read the instructions carefully first. In most cases you need to wash them a few times before use for optimum absorbency.
- With each brand ask:
  — How many nappies do you need to buy in total – does one size fit all?
  — What additional costs do you need to consider (e.g. reusable or disposable liners, waterproof covers)?
  — Will they fit toddlers until they are potty-trained?
  — How do you wash and dry them and how long do they take to dry?
- Brands to consider: Bambino Mio (Tel: 01604 458999), Bumkins (Tel: 0181 905 5661), Birthworks (Tel: 01364 72802), Earthwise Baby (Tel: 01908 585769 and available from Boots), Ellie Pants (Tel: 0151 200 5012), Galfies (Tel: 01428 682488 and independent stores), Kooshies (Tel: 0171 221 0041), Mikey Diaper (Tel: 0181 203 7122 and Mothercare), Poopers (Tel: 0161 777 9229), Sam I Am! (Tel: 0181 995 9204).

Using a Nappy Service
Nappy services supply you with a set of nappies and a deodorised nappy pail. They pick up your dirty nappies each week and replace them with clean ones. The cost is around £7–£9 a week, plus the cost of waterproof wraps. In total you may find this works out around the same as buying disposables but this method is generally considered the greener option.

If you want to check them out first:

- Ask to talk to existing customers about the service and check that they are reliable and that the nappies supplied are not too old.

- Ask if they will allow you a 'trial' period before committing to using the service long term.
- You may also want to check that the service follows Department of Health guidelines for sterilising nappies by washing them at a high temperature.
- Their delivery vans should have two different storage areas so that clean nappies cannot come into contact with dirty ones.
- You can contact NANS, the National Association of Nappy Services (Tel: 0121 693 4949), for details of a service in your area. NANS members wash and deliver nappies using preferred methods outlined above.

Changing Accessories

Shopping List
- Nappy rash cream.
- Muslin squares.
- Baby wipes.

Checklist
Nappy Rash Cream
- Sudocrem is at the top of most people's list, closely followed by other nappy rash creams from the chemist.
- Parents and carers also suggest: painting the affected area with egg white; letting your baby go without a nappy; and, after a bath, not rubbing the bottom dry but blow-drying it with a hair dryer.

Muslin Squares
- These are soft, thin and washable, and have multiple uses for all babies. Traditionally they are used as an inner lining on a terry nappy.
- Even if you do not use them for nappies, buy a pack. They are invaluable for: protecting your clothes while burping a baby, a soft bib for infants, an emergency changing mat, a sheet protector, pillow, sunshade, etc, etc.
- Muslin squares are also brilliant for laying over a plastic changing mat – then if the baby wees before you can get a new nappy on, it's soaked up by the muslin and the damage is limited.

Baby Wipes
For some reason, wipes often seem to be 'on special offer' or part of a 'two for the price of one' promotion. Many parents said that they usually bought the bargain. There was none of

the passionate brand loyalty that they expressed for nappies. Talking about nappies with one group, I really thought that two mothers were going to start hitting each other over the merits of Pampers v. Huggies.

Wipes usually come in square plastic tubs and these are the easiest to use. The square tubs are usually refillable and afterwards have hundreds of storage uses. They are ideal for small toys, crayons, etc.

Trying to extract wipes from a cylindrical tub while holding a baby is hard – you usually end up resembling an unwilling magician with a string of them flowing from your fingers. Refillable travel packs are also available and most people find them extremely useful for bottoms on the move.

Cheap wipes tend to be a false economy. They are so thin that you end up using far more than if you had used a thicker, seemingly pricier product.

Our nursery nurse panel tested a number of brands on a variety of bottoms but recommended only a few as follows.

Product Table

Baby Wipes	
Brand and Price	**Comments**
Boots Extra Soft Wipes (£2.99 for 80)	Needed one or two for each change; soft and sweet-smelling.
Johnson & Johnson (£3.49 for 80)	Needed two for each change. Loved the smell and the lotion feel.
Superdrug (£1.69 for 80)	Needed at least three per change but soft and moist.
Tesco (£2.09 for 84)	One or two per change; 'really nice, no need to rub, just wipe,' said our testers.
Pampers (£3.29 for 80)	Needed between one and three. Very soft.

Car Seats

The Child Accident Prevention Trust reckon that two-thirds of the children who are killed or hurt each year in cars would be saved by properly fitted restraints.

It is now illegal to either carry a baby in your arms in the car or to put a seat belt round yourself and a child. So, if you intend to drive your baby home from hospital, make sure that you are fully equipped in advance.

This is easier said than done but you will get it right if you follow the four rules:

- Don't buy any seat unless it fits your car perfectly.
- Base your choice on the weight of your baby rather than his age.
- Decide in advance if you want a seat that stays fixed in the car or a light portable one.
- Never put you baby in a seat with an airbag.

Shopping List

Seat size	Rough Age of Baby	Weight of Baby
0	Birth to around nine months	Up to 10kg (22lb)
0+	Birth to 12–15 months	Up to 13kg (29lb)
1	Around nine months to four years	9–18kg (20–40lb)
2	Around four to six years	15–25kg (33–55lb)
3	Around four to 11 years	15–36kg (33–79lb)

Once you know the size you need, choose a model (or two) from the following styles:

Sizes Available	Style of Car Seat
Size 0 Size 0+	*Infant carrier*, can be carried in and out of the car and allows a baby to sit facing the back of the seat. This is perceived as a particularly safe option.
Spans two sizes 0 and 1 or 0+ and 1	*Two-way seat.* If you buy the 0+ and 1 option, your baby will travel facing the back of the seat for longer than the 0 and 1 type.
Size 1 but some take children from size 1 to size 3	*Forward-facing seat with harness.*
Spans sizes 1 and 2. Some go from size 1 to size 3.	*Forward-facing seat without harness* (booster seat). Light and easy to move in and out of the car.

Checklist
What You Need to Know Before You Go Shopping

- Don't buy without trying it out first. If it doesn't fit perfectly into your car do not buy it.
- If you don't understand the manufacturer's fitting instructions, take the seat back. Find a seat that you can use easily.
- Most shops will not fit the seat for you as they could fall foul of their insurance cover if anything happened. What they tend to do is fit the seat, take it out and then watch you do it.
- Your baby's weight is the best indicator as to which size seat you need.
- The road safety officer at your local town hall may check your car seat over if you're worried; some do this for a small fee others for free.
- Some manufacturers offer new cars with integral baby car seats; these may be bolted into the car, limiting space for baby-free journeys. Check that this is not the case before you order.
- Never put a car seat near a passenger airbag. It could inflate, with fatal results.
- According to the latest research conducted by Renault, children in forward-facing seats are 20% more likely to be injured than those sitting in a backward-facing seat.

This may encourage you to look at 0+ seats which allow babies to face backwards until they are around nine months old (e.g. models such as the Rock a Tot and Bettacare Cygnet).

Parents' Choice for Newborns
In an ideal world, you would be 'better off buying an infant carrier which is as useful in the home as it is in the car,' say our families in Birmingham, a view echoed throughout most of the country. Another advantage is that if your baby has fallen asleep in the car, you can just carry him in and leave him to snooze in peace.

> *But watch your back.* Our researcher says that his chiropractor is alarmed by the number of mothers coming to see her because they have put their backs out by carrying baby seats using one arm. Try and spread the load by grasping the sides of the handles with both hands and carrying it in front of you.

The budget alternative
This is a two-way car seat which tends to be a hard-wearing, reasonably priced piece of kit that should last until your baby is around four years old. The drawback is that you cannot remove it easily from the car.

Once the Seat is in Use, Check
- The baby's harness is not too loose – you shouldn't be able to slip more than two fingers inside it.
- The adult seat belt is correctly routed and doesn't allow the seat to move around.
- The seat is replaced if it has been in a crash, even if it seems unscathed.
- The metal parts aren't too hot – they can heat up on sunny days and burn a baby.
- The belt buckle holding the child's seat in place isn't resting on the side of the seat frame as this pressure may force it open in a crash.

Stage 0 and Stage 0+ Car Seats/Infant Carriers

Baby's weight
Up to 10kg for size 0 car seats. Up to 13kg for size 0+ car seats.

Baby's age (approx)
Birth to between nine (size 0) and 15 (size 0+) months.

Position in car
Rearward-facing but do not use on front passenger seat if fitted with an airbag.

Fits into car
Using a standard adult seat belt.

Plus points
- Can be carried in and out of car without disturbing the baby.
- Useful at home as a baby seat.
- Can be bought as part of a buggy travel system (see pp. 126–7).

Minus point
Only lasts until the baby reaches 13kg (maximum with a 0+ size).

Signs that your baby needs a bigger seat
- He has reached the weight limit.
- He can sit up for long periods without support.
- His head is higher than the seat.

Two-way Seats
These stay put in the car and so lack a handle like the infant carrier but will fit most children until they weigh 18kg and are around four years old. They face rearwards initially and become forward facing once the baby can hold his head up.

Three-way Seats
These are designed to last from birth up to six years old. They are new on the market in 1999 so we have been unable to test

them prior to publication. They should be considered as they represent excellent value and minimal hassle as you only have to make one purchase.

Stage 2 Car Seats

Baby's weight
From 15kg up to 25kg (33lb to 55lb).

Baby's age (approx)
Four to six years.

Position in car
Forward facing (do not use on seat fitted with an air-bag).

Fits into car
Using adult seat belt or special fixing kit.

Plus points
- Provide good sideways protection.
- Are often easy to fit.
- Can be reclined for long journeys.

Minus points
- Not many models to choose from, as stage 3 seats are more popular.
- Can be hefty and are unsuitable for moving from car to car.
- Models without five-point harnesses may allow your child to slip out easily but some children suss all harness mechanisms in a few seconds anyway.

Signs that your child needs a bigger seat
- He has reached the weight limit.
- His eye level is above the back of the seat.

Stage 3 Car Seats/Booster Seats

Child's weight
Can be up to 36kg (79lb), depending on model chosen.

Child's age (approx)
Up to seven years old, depending on model.

Position in car
Faces forward (do not use on a seat fitted with an air-bag).

Fits into car
Using standard car seat belt.

Plus points
- Portable and good value — ideal for moving from one car to another.
- Easy to sling in the boot when not in use.

Minus points
Some models aren't supportive enough for younger children. The child must be able to sit unsupported before using these seats.

Product Table

It's difficult to make particular recommendations as the most important thing is to find a seat that fits your car. However, we couldn't resist highlighting a few really popular and very good-value seats.

Infant Carriers

Model	Price	Weight	Comments
For babies weighing 0–10kg (up to 22lb) or 0–13kg (up to 29lb)			
Britax Rock a Tot ☺	£59.99	0–13kg	Absolute favourite – great for low-birthweight babies. Can be used in the Britax Travel System.
Klippan Carry One Plus	£49.99	0–13kg	Easy fold handle, integral storage box, headhugger included in price.
Jeenay Nest 'N' Rest £	£20	0–10kg	Very light, good for parents of multiples. A real bargain.

CAR SEATS

Infant Carriers (continued)

Model	Price	Weight	Comments
Bettacare Cygnet ☺	£47.99	0–13kg	Excellent for low-birthweight babies. Has performed well in consumer tests and good value considering how long you can use it.

Helplines: Britax (01264 333343), Klippan (01228 535544), Bettacare (01293 851896), Cosatto (01268 727070), Jeenay (0121 327 1422). Mamas and Papas now carry a range of seats. If you have an M&P pram, you may want to buy their car seat that clips onto the pram chassis – see Travel Systems on pp. 127–132 or ring M&P (01484 438222).

Car Seats

Model	Price	Comments
***Two-way Seats** – for newborn to around four years old (up to 18kg or 40lb)*		
Britax Club Class ☺	£110	One-pull tensioning. Twin belt system. Five reclining positions. Padded, machine-washable covers. Raised seat allows babies to see out of the window. Play tray (£10.75) available as an extra.
Cosatto GoSafe Evolution	£99.99	One-pull tensioning. Five reclining positions but check out the harness – may prove fiddly.
Black leather 'Sports Deluxe'	£300	Padded, machine-washable covers or black leather.
Jeenay Guardian Platinum £	£64.99	One-pull tensioning. Padded covers – hand wash only. Heavy for moving around and difficult to recline with baby in situ. Has additional head and shoulder pads. Raised seat allows babies to see out of the window. But a great price.
***Forward-facing Seats with Harness** – for around nine months to four years old (9–18kg; 20–40lb)*		
Britax Freeway Excel 03 ☺	£99.99	One-pull harness; washable covers; one reclining position. Play tray available as an extra (£10.75).

Car Seats (continued)

Model	Price	Comments
Klippan Premier Plus	£90	One-pull harness, good side support and multi-position recline but small for a growing child.
Maxi Cosi Priori	£119	Five-position recline; one-pull harness; marginally smaller than Britax seat. Many people buy this if their child hates the car as side hooks for the harness keep it out of the way. This means that when he goes rigid and shrieks in your face, you don't have to scrabble under his bottom for the belt.
Mothercare Venturer	£89.99	One-pull harness; multi-position recline; machine-washable covers. Footrest for additional comfort.
Mothercare Little Trekker	£49.99	If your child is on the petit side consider this. Although it seems less substantial and smaller than other models, it still meets the stringent British Standard and it is less than half the price of most other seats around.

Forward-facing Seat without Harness – for babies weighing from 9kg (20lb) to between 25kg and 36kg (55–79lb)

Model	Price	Comments
Britax Super-Cruiser	£59.99	For children from 9–25kg. A wonderful seat that can be moved from car to car or put in the boot with minimal fuss.
Britax Javelin	£89.99	For children from 9–36kg. As above but base detaches to give a booster seat for children up to 11. In practice, a larger child may not need a booster and if you buy a new car during the next 10 years the booster may not fit anyway. You can always buy one separately later.

Car Seat Accessories

You can kiss goodbye to the joys of the open road. Car journeys will never be the same again, now that your car is a livestock container – complete with noise, smell and mess.

Many parents report that they have become so used to distracting infant passengers that years later they are still shrieking with excitement 'Ooh look there's a horsey!', much to the surprise of clients or colleagues who happen to be in the car at the time.

Everybody has different ways of coping with their children on car journeys. Food and drink will usually shut them up but it will also go everywhere. Well-designed equipment should minimise the chaos but the only failsafe method – a gag and a straitjacket (for your kids during the trip and yourself after it) – must contravene at least 10 EC regulations.

Below is a choice of goods designed to make your car trips less painful.

Product Table

Equipment/Toys for Car Travel	
Product, Price and Stockists	**Comments**
Rear-Seat Mirrors – allow drivers to see back-seat passengers without turning round.	
JoJo Child Mirror (£3.99)	This clips to your rear-view mirror or you can use the windscreen suction pad.
Boots Child View Mirror (£5 – Mail order: 0845 840 1000)	A small circular mirror that you fix onto your windscreen below your rear-view mirror.

Equipment/Toys for Car Travel (continued)

Product, Price and Stockists	Comments
Panoramic Rear-View Mirror (£7.99) Great Little Trading Company	An oversized rear-view mirror that removes blind spots outside the car, with a smaller mirror attached below so you can see the back seat.
Car Sunshades	
Mothercare Retractable Sunblind (£5.99 – Mail order: 01923 240365)	This attaches to the car window using either suction pads or clips and rolls up when not in use.
Mothercare Car Sunscreen (£4.99)	As above but cannot be rolled up.
JoJo (set of two for £5.99)	Bargain pop-open shades that fold down to 10cm for easy storage.
In-Car Entertainment and Storage	
Car Bar (£16.99) + Car Bar Phone (£7.99) + Bottle Holder – JoJo	An activity bar made of soft fabric; includes a steering wheel and toy. Extras (priced separately) can be attached.
Car Toy Box (£12.99) Great Little Trading Company	Organiser bag – attaches to seat-belt clip.
Car Litter Container (£9.99) Great Little Trading Company	Fits onto back of front seat and closes neatly to hide rubbish inside.
Backpocket (£9.99) Great Little Trading Company	Three-layered mesh pockets on a backing. Installation as above.
Activity Play Tray (£14.99) Mothercare	Features a squeaky soft steering wheel.
In-Car Food and Drink Storage	
Car Snack Tray (£4.99) JoJo	Hooks onto door and takes a cup and a snack.
Car Bottle Cooler (£4.99) JoJo	Sucker attaches cooler to window.
Boots Car Tray (£12.99)	Larger than above, this fits onto back of front seat and folds away when not in use.

Equipment/Toys for Car Travel (continued)

Product, Price and Stockists	Comments
Sleep Cushions – to stop child's head lolling forward if he falls asleep in the car.	
Nap 'N' Go from Safety First (£3.99)	

For music and story tapes, see p. 168.

> Don't allow a small baby to eat while the car is moving or give him toys that you think he may be tempted to throw at the driver. Instead, you can buy a Car Activity Centre (£9.99 from Blooming Marvellous mail order) or a soft fabric activity play tray (£17.99 from Tesco Direct).

Pushchairs and Buggies

'Buggy' is used as a generic term when discussing wheeled goods in these introductory pages.

Not only is this a seriously expensive item of babygear but if you make a mistake you will be reminded of it every time you see the wretched thing lurking by the front door . . . if you can get it through the door at all! This will be one of your most important purchases and most people get it wrong because they are attracted to pretty fabric rather than sturdy design.

But never fear – *The Best Baby Buys Guide* will help you find your way through the minefield. Just don't let the buggies get you down!

Shopping List
For a Newborn Baby – One of the Following:
- A pram – a traditional conveyance with a flat bed.
- A convertible pushchair (also called a two-in-one) – a reclining seat unit that can lie flat when your baby is small and become a pushchair later. A two-in-one-plus allows a seat unit to be lifted off the chassis and used as a carrycot.
- A combination 'combo' pushchair (also called a three-in-one) – a two-in-one with a carrycot included in the price.
- A fully reclining buggy/stroller – usually more lightweight and easier to fold than the models above. Suitable for use from birth.
- A travel system – a two-in-one or three-in-one, as above, which comes with a car seat that will slot onto the pushchair chassis.
- A buggy/stroller.

For Two Children (Twins or Siblings) – One of the Following:
- A fully reclining twin pushchair.

- A tandem pushchair.
- A pushchair/buggy with a platform for the older child to stand on.

Optional Accessories for All Models
- Sun canopy.
- Foot muff/cosytoes.
- Co-ordinating changing bag.
- PVC waterproof cover.

My Personal View
As the choice of buggies can leave you feeling dizzy, this is the only chapter where I am venturing to give a very personal opinion. Bearing in mind that I dislike walking, love the car and am city-based, I would choose either a travel system (see pp. 125–130) or a fully reclining, umbrella-fold buggy (see p. 131) that is suitable from birth.

Most people come to an umbrella-fold stroller once they are heartily sick of lugging their bulkier 'designer' model around, but why waste the initial hundreds of pounds when you can go straight to the umbrella option? If you have to have a more traditional model incorporating a carrycot for the first few weeks you can borrow or rent one. I was quoted £35 a month for a top-quality buggy with a carrycot by Jack and Jill in Leeds (freephone: 0800 026 9370). For details of over 100 hire firms nationally, ring the Babyline (Tel: 0831 310355). I always seem to ring when the phone is being charged but I'm sure that's just my timing.

If I lived in a rural environment, I might go for an easy-folding buggy offering good protection and big wheels; an all-terrain model suitable from birth if I was sporty; and a travel system if I wasn't.

Traditionalists may throw up their hands in horror at this view, saying that a baby needs to lie totally flat on a proper mattress. But consider how long your baby will be in the buggy for. If you are a driver, the answer is probably an hour at most on a normal day. The rest of the day, your baby can lie on a mattress – in his cot or Moses basket.

If you are expecting twins or more, get advice from your local Twins Club (number available from Tamba, see p. 13).

Checklist – Before You Go Shopping
Consider Your Home

- Measure the width of your doorway. Your buggy must fit through it easily. Otherwise, every time you arrive home with your baby, you will end up having to wake him, then carry the baby under one arm, your buggy under the other and your shopping in your jaws. (Now you know why all the women in pram advertisements are either talking to their partners through clenched teeth or are using mobile phones – 'Sorry to interrupt your board meeting, darling, but I can't get this bloody pram into the house . . .')
- Decide where your buggy will be stored when it is not in use. Make sure that you choose a model that will fit the area available – ideally somewhere near the front door.
- If you will be wheeling your buggy up and down stairs, restrict your choice to lighter models.

Consider the Demands of Your Lifestyle

- If you will need to fold your buggy into your car, measure the dimensions of your car boot, remembering that you will need to allow space for both the buggy and other luggage.
- If you are a walker and will rarely put your buggy in your car, you will want good suspension and maybe larger wheels.
- If you have set your heart on a larger model, make sure that you have enough storage space for it.
- For shopping, a large, low shopping tray is essential, even if all you want to transport is your baby's changing bag. It is dangerous to hang bags from the handle.
- If your buggy will be used by a number of different people (grandparents, childminders, etc), simplicity is all-important. You don't want someone accidentally collapsing the buggy with your baby in it or catching your baby's fingers while they wrestle with the folding mechanism. Adjustable handles will also be useful.

Consider Cost and Quality

- Decide on a budget and stick to it. More expensive does not necessarily mean better quality. You may not need all

the special features on offer. And, with some models, there are hidden extras that may not be included in the original price quoted to you. Make sure you know exactly what is included, rather than receiving a nasty shock when you pick up your order six weeks later.
- Check that it conforms to BS 7409:1996. The label will usually be found under the seat.
- Consider the length of time you will use it for. If you are buying any form of convertible or combination buggy, for example, concentrate on the pushchair option, as this will be in use far longer than the lie-flat/carrycot. As most families end up relying on a light, space-saving umbrella-fold buggy, you may want to allow for this in your pram budget.
- Consider buying overseas. You may find a seemingly identical product overseas at a better price (exchange rates permitting). A few people we spoke to had ordered equipment from the USA or had gone on a buggy-buying trip to France and were thrilled with their purchases. Go for it – but remember that it may not meet the strenuous British Standard BS 7409:1996. (This requires buggies to have linked brakes. But these are not standard in the EEC. In Europe, many buggies have just the one brake. When parked on a slope, this means the pram can still swivel round on its non-braking wheels.)

For Product Tables for two-in-ones, three-in-ones, travel systems and strollers, see pp. 127–131. For double buggies, twin strollers and tandems, see p. 134. For all-terrain buggies, see pp. 135–136.

Checklist – in the Shop
Safety
- Only consider reputable brands with a proper guarantee.
- Fatalities can occur with buggies. Don't take a chance with shoddy goods.

Shopping Around
- Some retailers have built up relationships with particular manufacturers and can offer discounts.

- Because buggies are now 'fashion' items, you may find a sale bargain – if you don't mind last year's fabric.

Trusting Your Own Instincts
- We spoke to many parents who regretted their pram purchase and admitted that they had based their choice either on stylish looks or the fact that 'everyone else seemed to have the same'.
- The other cause of grief was mother-in-laws who insisted on buying their own idea of a great pram.
- As your best friends will tell you – performance is all-important. Looks are secondary.

Choosing Another Fabric
- If you dislike the colourway shown on your preferred model ask if they have samples of alternative fabrics or look at the product catalogue. (These are available from the numbers listed on pp. 121–2, as well as from most retailers.) There may well be more attractive choices that are being suppressed while they try to shift the uglier ones.

After-Sales Care
- If the buggy has a problem can they mend it on site?
- If it is sent away for repairs will they lend you another one?

Weight and Size
- Lift it up to get a good idea of the weight.
- The labelling on different prams and buggies can be misleading, as it doesn't always compare like with like. For example, one pram might show the weight of the chassis plus carrycot but another might indicate the weight of the chassis alone.
- Take a tape measure with you. And, if you are concerned that your preferred buggy will not fit into the car boot or your home, measure the size both open and closed.

Folding Mechanisms
- Some buggies fold flat; some are free-standing in a folded position. Some need two hands to fold; some only one. Ideally you want one that works easily with just one hand, as you may be holding your baby with the other.
- If you go to a nursery store with a car park outside, the assistants may let you try folding different models into your car boot.

The Wheels and Suspension
- Larger wheels are best for suspension. Swivel wheels are essential for shopping or on double buggies, as they remove the need to lever the pram round corners. Large, fixed wheels are better for rough surfaces.
- Test the suspension before you buy. Wheel it round the shop a few times to see how it feels.

The Seat
- If you are buying a conveyance for a newborn, the seat must fully recline. Otherwise, a number of reclining options are worth having for a buggy that is in constant use. A single-position seat is fine for holiday use.
- A reversible seat unit allows the baby to face towards you in the early months and away from you later on. Some researchers said that they felt it was important to choose a buggy in which your baby was facing you during his early weeks. Some good-value models don't have this feature. They may have a window in the hood so that you can see your baby but the problem is – he can't see you.

The Shopping Tray
- Grab a pack of nappies off the shelf and see if it fits in the tray with room to spare.

The Handle
- Check that it suits you, if your partner is very tall and you are very short.
- Some brands, e.g. Bebe Confort, offer adjustable handle heights.

The Harness
- Your buggy should come with a five-point harness. If it does not, buy one and use it.

Buying Second-Hand Wheeled Goods (Buggies, Prams, etc)
- It should not be rusty.
- Neither the frame nor the handle should be bent.
- Folding parts should move smoothly.
- Locks should be in perfect condition and not be able to collapse while the buggy is in use.
- Tears in the seat or the fabric make a buggy potentially dangerous and difficult to clean.
- Wheels must be in perfect alignment, touching the ground equally and not worn in odd places.
- Wobbly wheels may suggest that the bearings need to be replaced – a potentially expensive repair.
- The brakes must work perfectly – even when you push hard on the buggy.

See pp. 8–12 for general advice on buying second-hand goods.

Buggy Accessories Checklist
Sun Canopy
- As the sun always seems to find a way round a canopy or parasol, a hat, sun-screen and protective clothing are probably more reliable.
- If you want to be absolutely sure that not a single ray hits your baby, buy a canopy but do not neglect to keep his skin protected as well.
- Parasols tend to be less robust than canopies.

Foot Muff/Cosytoes
- Not one person has suggested these as a top buy but they are often included in the price of a buggy.
- They're certainly not essential – if your baby is dressed warmly that should be sufficient.

PVC Waterproof Cover
- Our researcher in the Scottish Highlands thought this a 'must' while our ladies in London thought them a waste of money. In short, if you are walking through the heather on a daily basis there is no other way to shelter your baby in a downpour. If you are in a city centre and can pop into a nice little café when it pours – why bother? See how you get on without one, before shelling out.
- For waterproof snowsuits, see pp. 22–23.

When to Buy Accessories

You used to have to buy all your accessories at the same time as you bought your buggy to ensure that they would fit and co-ordinate.

If you want a sun canopy in co-ordinating fabric, you may still have to do this. But, if you're not that bothered and want to wait and see if you really need any of the products listed above, you can be guaranteed of a product that will fit by buying the Ninaclip range. If you buy the rain cover (£9.99 – basic, £15.99 – lie-back), you will get two clips into which you can also click your Nina Parasol (£15.99) or your Nina Canopy (£19.99).

Each product comes with its own clip in the pack but they fit any buggy, so if you have a spare buggy for holidays you can easily transfer your accessories from one to the other. Spare clips cost £5.99 for two.

Contacting Pram Manufacturers

To contact pram manufacturers, ring the following telephone numbers.

Babysphere:	01788 544600
Bébécar:	0181 201 0505
Bébé Confort:	01484 401802
Britax:	01264 386034
Chicco:	01623 750870
Cossatto:	01268 452288

Emmaljunga:	0116 260 5966
Graco:	0870 909 0510
Maclaren:	01327 842662
Mamas and Papas:	01484 438226
Monbebe:	01484 401100
Mothercare:	01923 210210
Silver Cross:	0800 731 7689
Waki:	01895 812256

Prams

These are suitable from birth to around eight months. They should reach BS 7409:1996.

A pram is a large, flat bed with a big-wheeled chassis, giving magnificent suspension. They are a joy to push. And, although there are other brands around, none have the cachet of Silver Cross. It is rare to find a retailer stocking anything else.

Unlike the more modern combination and convertible prams, they are bulky to store and heavy to transport. But, if that doesn't bother you, you can choose between the classic 'coach-built' prams with steel sides and the fabric models. The hard-bodied ones can be wiped clean. The soft-bodied ones are spongeable.

Note: Pram sheets are a waste of money. Just fold your cot sheets to fit.

Reasons for Caution
- A pram is an expensive purchase, especially as it will only be used for a matter of months and you will then have to buy something else. Look for mattresses 84cm long, as they will be in use longer than the 78cm-length models.
- You will need space to store it and no front steps. The superior models are too large and heavy to be hauled up steps by a new mother. They were designed with a good, strong nanny in mind.
- Larger prams are not appropriate for daily car travel. Although wheels are generally removable for transportation, big prams are still relatively cumbersome to collapse and carry around.
- Larger prams may prove awkward in shops. There is no way that you could manoeuvre one of these into a Kookai changing cubicle.

Product Table

All models are detailed in the Silver Cross Catalogue (Tel: 0800 731 7689). Last year there were 11 to choose from, three of which appear in the table below. Stork Talk (Tel: 0115 930 6700) often have 'bargain' Silver Cross prams available and will deliver them to your door.

Prams				
Model and Price	Age	Gross Weight	Bed Size (cm)	Comments
In all the following models the shopping tray comes as an extra, costing £20.				
Silver Cross Marlborough (£499)	Birth+	34kg	85×36×17	Steel-bodied, traditional pram. Not for disassembly.
Silver Cross Windsor (£365)	Birth+	25kg	78×36×19	Steel-bodied with folding chassis and removable wheels but still an armful to throw in the car boot.
Silver Cross Marquis (£240)	Birth+	23kg	84×39×19	Soft-bodied with folding chassis. The cheapest and lightest but with a better-sized bed than many.

Convertibles, Combinations and Travel Systems

I've been standing in a branch of John Lewis for 45 minutes indulging in a new spectator sport – a team event for sales assistants opening and closing numerous combination prams in the fastest possible time. Can't you just see it – Olympic synchronised buggy-collapsing, with points awarded for style and technical merit.

These assistants gave me the impression that they were having such fun performing buggy weight-training for an appreciative audience that they did not necessarily want to recommend the simplest, best-value conveyance – which is what we actually need. 'Never knowingly understood' should be their new slogan.

Sales staff are not necessarily bothered by the many factors that should govern this expensive purchase. In fact, a test of a good shop is how many questions they ask you about your domestic and travelling requirements before they start demonstrating various buggy models.

When you decide on your preferred model, you should leave the store feeling absolutely confident that you can use your combination buggy in any form, in any situation.

I'm telling you this because of the number of parents who told us that they really regretted their choice. Don't let yourself be swayed by visions of yourself performing pram aerobics for the neighbours. You must be certain of what you need before you cross any palms with plastic.

Checklist

Two-in-One Convertibles

- This is a pushchair seat that reclines to form a fully enclosed carrycot-type bed. This is smaller than a real carrycot and you cannot lift the unit off the chassis (though there are exceptions, like the two-in-one-plus – see Product Table opposite).
- When the convertible is being used as a pushchair, you can alter the position of the seat unit and most chairs can be positioned either facing outwards or facing the carer.
- These are a good idea if you are buying a car seat separately (if not, see Travel Systems, below and pp. 129–130).
- You can also wheel a convertible indoors to use as a day bed for your baby (though the beds tend to be small and narrow).
- The suspension is not usually that good, although you will probably have a choice of wheel types.

Three-in-One Combinations (or 'Combos')

- These have all the advantages of the two-in-one plus a proper-sized carrycot.
- Prices are often comparable to a two-in-one but you get more for your money.
- The seat unit is removable to allow the carrycot to be attached to the chassis. This creates a proper-sized pram unit on buggy wheels.
- A carrycot can be used instead of a Moses basket as a baby bed.
- Adaptor kits are available to allow carrycots to be anchored safely to a car seat. While in the car, your baby must wear a harness for safety.

Travel Systems

- A travel system is a pushchair with clips for a size 0 (birth–10kg) car seat. You can lift the car seat straight out of the car and clip it onto the pushchair chassis without having to disturb your baby.
- With some brands (like Century and Maclaren), the pushchair seat remains on the chassis and the car seat slots on top. This can look strange.

- A given travel system will only take one specific model of car seat, made by the pushchair manufacturer. If that model does not fit well in your car do not buy it.
- A travel system is a good bet if you want an infant carrier/first car seat.
- It's also a good option if your car boot is too small to take anything more than a chassis.
- They tend to be very light.
- Most paediatricians say that it is not a good idea to keep a baby sitting in a car seat for long periods. They are better off lying on their backs in a more unrestricted environment. A travel system combo comes with a carry-cot as well, so, should you go for a walk, you can still push your baby around in a more traditional manner.

Strollers

- Most strollers are umbrella-folding models – they tend to be the cheapest, lightest, most convenient option.
- They're excellent if you have limited storage space.
- And they're ideal for travelling.
- Even if you have an amazing combination buggy, you can get a basic umbrella-folding stroller for only £20 at Mothercare which is ideal for holidays and keeping in the car boot.

Product Table

Two-in-Ones (Convertibles)

Model, Price and Weight	Extras Included in Price	Comments
Babysphere Apollo (£499) Weight of seat and chassis combined: 9kg	Hood, rain cover, parasol and cosytoes	This convertible is particularly expensive because it includes a battery-driven filtration unit that removes 98% of air pollutants (not tested).

Two-in-Ones (Convertibles) (continued)

Model, Price and Weight	Extras Included in Price	Comments
Cosatto Volante (£389) Weight of seat and chassis combined: 14.2kg	Hood and apron	A traditional model with all the features you could hope for and an adjustable handle and good-looking bed option. Seat reverses to face pusher.
Maclaren Clio (£219) Weight of seat and chassis combined: 11.9kg	Hood, apron and shopping tray	Incredible value for a versatile product. On buggy wheels. Seat reverses to face pusher.
Mothercare Sorrento (£229) Weight of seat and chassis combined: 9.2kg	Hood, apron and shopping tray	A lightweight product which 'gives you the convenience of a stroller while your baby has the comfort of a pushchair'.

Mamas and Papas do a number of models that are worth checking out. The Sherpa Streetwise is both sporty and great value at £220, the Plikomatic Elegante is £210, and the Pliko Sportivo is £190. All have designs and features that will appeal to the fussiest of purchasers. But they are not cheap.

Emmaljunga is another brand that is worth looking at. All their products are wonderfully made – modern materials upholding traditional designs.

Three-in-One Combinations

Model and Price	Age	Pushchair/Buggy Weight	Comments
All the following models include reversible seat, carrycot and shopping tray.			
Mamas and Papas Carlotta on classic chassis (£445)	Birth+	11kg	Retailers love this model, presumably because its good looks ensure lots of sales. But you have to pay for extras like the canopy.
Mamas and Papas Combi Streetwise on Sherpa chassis (£399)	Birth+	10kg	A sporty version but, again, beware the cost of extras, e.g. the canopy (£29.95).
Bébé Confort Grand Style Chassis: £160 Carrycot: £190 Seat unit: £90	Birth+	10.5kg	A wonderful-quality product that will really last but you cannot use the hood or apron from the carrycot with the seat unit.
Silver Cross Chaser (£309)	Birth+	15kg	This will be your mother-in-law's choice, but it's a heavy option.

Travel Systems

Model and Price	Carrycot	Comments
Graco Denver Travel System (£219) £	N/A	Amazing value; efficient model adored by press. But, as car seat locks into pushchair seat, rather than straight onto chassis, it looks rather clumsy. The seat does not reverse to face pusher and shopping tray may be tricky to access when the seat is lying flat.

Travel Systems (continued)

Model and Price	Carrycot	Comments
Bébé Confort Limousine Chassis and pushchair (£210) Car seat (£70) Fixing kit (£10) ♛	Prelude £170 with fixing can be used for car travel	Expensive but excellent quality. Possibly worth considering if you are planning a tribe. Seat reverses to face pusher.
Britax Trio Travel System (£239) + Rock a Tot car seat ☺	N/A	The Rock a Tot car seat is a firm favourite and the pushchair is good and sturdy, although it does not go totally flat in the newborn position. Seat reverses to face pusher.
Bébécar Travel System. Chassis: £130 Car seat: £110	Pushchair unit and separate carrycot: £260	You can choose from a range of different chassis designs and match them to interchangeable units. Hood, apron and waterproof coverall included in price. Seat reverses to face pusher.
Mamas and Papas 'Classic' Chassis: £175 Pushchair and carrycot (one unit): £255 Uni-Traveller car seat: £54.95	Yes but price in first column for two-in-one and convertible unit	As some readers will only consider a Mamas and Papas buggy, it's worth noting that their Uni-Traveller car seat will fit onto any Mamas and Papas pushchair chassis. Seat reverses to face pusher.

Strollers

Model and Price	Age	Comments
Graco 'Mirage' (£99) £	0+ (seat reclines to 15° off flat)	A worldwide bestseller. Not an umbrella-folding model but does fold flat. Offers a newborn lots of padding and protection. Huge shopping basket.
Maclaren Opus V (£180) ☺	0+ (fully reclining)	New and impressive umbrella-folding model from the reliable Maclaren stable. Comes with shopping basket, hood and footmuff. Raincover is £20.50 extra.
Maclaren Free Spirit (£179)	0+ (fully reclining)	Another new umbrella-folding Maclaren. This is 'designed to protect on the roughest terrain'. We were unsure about the spongy handles but otherwise found it a joy. Shopping basket comes as an extra but rucksack changing bag is included.
Maclaren Micra (£29.99)	Six months (for babies able to sit up unaided)	Perfect holiday buggy. One position, umbrella-folding, weighs 5.3kg, but has swivel wheels and is well made.
Bébé Confort Laser (£99.95) ☺	0+	Excellent, unusual umbrella-folding model with good recline. Includes basket. Reliably informed that it fits in the boot of a Porsche. Weighs only 6kg.

Double Buggies

If you are expecting twins or more, you will want a double buggy. But, if you are thinking of getting a buggy to seat an older and younger child, think twice. This can end up being very heavy – at times you will have to lever up the combined weight of the children and buggy. The weight and awkwardness of using one of these can hurt your back so be careful how you push.

If your children don't get on well, or one bullies the other, side-by-sides in particular are torture for the weaker child. He is held firmly in place by the five-point harness while being thoroughly thumped by his fellow passenger.

Alternatives to a Double Buggy
These include a single buggy for the older child and a sling for the baby, or a platform that attaches to the buggy for the older child to stand on. Or you might consider a Waki Le Shuttle. This comes with an integral platform for the older child to stand on, and costs £159.99 (+£29.99 extra for the babykit to make the seat suitable for use by a newborn baby).

Checklist
Side-by-Sides

- The babies sit next to each other. This means that they can both recline and you can see what they are both up to.
- Wider models are not ideal for shopping as you may not be able to fit through a doorway and some do not have shopping trays.
- The advantage of a side-by-side is that they are usually easier to manoeuvre than a tandem.
- All-terrain versions are available. Contact Pegasus (Tel: 01822 618077).

Tandems
- The babies sit one in front of the other.
- These are as slim as a single buggy and there is usually room for a large shopping tray.
- But, to some, they seem heavier than a side-by-side and their length makes them tricky to push.
- They also tend to be harder to fold into a car boot.

General Features
- You will need fully reclining seats for newborns. (Not all 'newborn' models lie completely flat.)
- Narrower buggies are easier to get through doorways but wider ones will accommodate growing bottoms and should last longer.
- If you are dependent on a lift to get to your front door, check that the buggy will fit inside it.
- If you need a transportable model, check that it will fit in your boot.
- Check that the buggy has lockable swivel wheels.
- Separate seats allow one to be reclined while the other stays upright but some twins like the security of being close to each other on a single bench seat. Take advice from your local twins club (or the Tamba twinline: 01732 868000).
- You will need five-point harnesses.
- Check whether accessories (e.g. shopping baskets) are included in the price.
- You must be able to open, close and adjust the buggy in moments.

Product Table

What we looked for:

- Reasonable weight and width.
- Folded size.
- Ease of use.
- Comfort.

Twin Strollers and Tandems

Model and Price	Age	Comments
Note: All of these should fit through a standard doorway.		
Graco Duo Literider from Babies 'R' Us and independent retailers (£179) £	0+ (seat reclines to 15° off flat)	Folds flat. Offers newborns individual seats and lots of padding and protection. Huge shopping basket. A bargain. Weight: 8kg. A similar product, at the same price, called a Twin Mirage, is sold in Mothercare.
Mamas and Papas Twin Micro Coperta (£239)	0+	Slim and glamorous; free-standing when folded with useful integral rain canopy. Has a white footrest. Would have thought anything white was a bit of a no-no! Has a carrying strap for easy lugging about. Shopping basket is an extra. Weight: 9.5kg.
Maclaren Mistral Duo (£129) £	Six months+	Looks pretty basic but is both light and well made, making it ideal for older, heavier twins. Weight: 9.4kg. Shopping basket comes as an extra.
Maclaren Duette (£159) ☺	0+	Lots of twins clubs recommend these and the fact that you can get a perfectly good one second-hand tells you what a good-quality buy it is. But, at 11.2kg, it's the heaviest of the favourites. Shopping basket is an extra.

We did not receive one parent-of-twins' endorsement of a tandem, possibly because they start at around £200 and weigh 12kg or more. Parents with babies of different ages liked the very solid Emmaljunga 'Grizzly' (£215), a buggy with a toddler chair (£52.95) attached. The Silver Cross Wayfarer is also worth checking out, although it can prove too bulky for some.

All-Terrain Buggies

The deeply trendy all-terrain buggy (as pushed by Tom Cruise) has a hammock-like seat and three large, fixed wheels. These buggies are usually bought in addition to a more orthodox conveyance.

Checklist
- You will need a huge car boot – some of these are tricky to fold down.
- An all-terrain buggy is great if you want to jog behind it – they are specially designed so you won't trip on the frame as you run.
- They're also a good bet if you want to wheel your baby across rugged countryside or sandy beaches.
- Check whether or not the shopping basket and sun canopy are included – they can add quite a bit to the price.

Product Table
What we looked for:

- Models that would suit a variety of needs.
- Ease of use – simple to open and collapse.
- Durability.
- Useful extras included in the price.
- Value for money.

All-Terrain Buggies

Model, Price and Stockists	Weight	Comments
Note: All of these models have a seat recline and are suitable for babies who can sit up unaided.		
Mountain Buggy (£325 including delivery) Stockists (Tel: 01276 502587)	9kg	Best for shopping – good big basket. Sun canopy included in price. Can be adapted for newborns by buying a hammock (£40).
Omni All-Terrain Buggy (£199 including delivery) Tel: 01727 811221	9 kg	The bargain buy. All extras included in price. Can be adapted for newborns. Designed for jogging as well as hiking. Should fit easily into the boot of a Micra.
Pegasus Trecker (£270) and Land Rover (£392) Well illustrated in Urchin catalogue (Tel: 01672 872872). Or ring direct on 01822 618077 for 200 local stockists	5.9kg	For the true all-terrain parent, Pegasus is the brand of choice. Some models include extras and others don't. Choose a combination to suit your needs and budget. Newborn cot seat available.

Holidays with a Baby

One response on this subject (from a mother of three) was: 'You've seen those circus vans on the motorway – well that's what it's like. Just *don't do it*! Forget it!'

The logistics of 'baby comes too' trips are enough to engender a new illness – Pre-Traumatic Stress Syndrome. Even before you've left the house, you will probably have assembled a mountain of luggage 10 times the size of the baby it belongs to. But, as any Girl Guide will tell you, you have to 'Be Prepared' to get the most out of a challenging situation.

If you forget an essential that you have to buy at your destination, don't let that carefree holiday feeling blind you to making careful choices. A dangerous product could ruin not only your holiday but your child's life.

Packing List

Note: What you take with you depends on individual circumstances but it might be worth asking your travel agent what will be available at your destination.

- Feeding equipment (see below).
- Bibs (see pp. 215–216).
- Travel highchair for larger babies (see pp. 219–220).

Breastfed Babies

- Breast pump (see pp. 62–64).
- Bottles for feeding breast milk (see pp. 36–42).
- Steriliser – optional (see pp. 43–47).

Bottle-fed Babies

- Disposable bottles (see p. 42).
- Formula dispensers (see p. 49).

- Travel bottles (see p. 49).
- Steriliser, as above.
- Cartons of ready-to-serve formula.

Babies on Solids
- Jars of food (see p. 208).
- Anyway-up-cup or similar (see pp. 213–214).
- Sealable food containers (see p. 209).
- Bowl and spoon (see pp. 212–213).
- Baby clothes – take plenty of clothes so you don't have to wash them every day.
- Nappies (see pp. 94–97).
- Baby wipes (see p. 102).
- Baby bath (see pp. 32–33).
- Umbrella-fold buggy (see p. 131) – you can usually wheel these right up to the plane door. Some models fit into overhead lockers but you may have a job persuading the cabin crew to let you bring it in. In which case they put it in the hold as you board and you collect it at the gate or off the luggage carousel at your destination.
- Toys and books – take ones that your children won't mind losing.
- Sun hat, protective clothing and suncreeen for hot destinations (see Product Table on pp. 143–144).
- Swimming aids (see pp. 145–146).
- Any large bag (preferably waterproof) for easy access to nappies, feeds, toys.
- Sling or backpack (see pp. 153–157).
- Travel cot (see pp. 199–201).
- Adaptor plug – if you are taking steriliser or baby monitor.
- First aid box, including Calpol, insect repellent and rehydration salts (see pp. 87–88).
- If you are travelling overseas, your baby must be included on your passport. Babies will need their own passport if they are not already included on that of their parents.
- Form E111 from the Post Office entitles you to free medical treatment in EC countries but not everything is covered so you may need additional travel insurance.

What You Will Need on the Journey

Assume that wherever you're going, you will be delayed. Pack hand-luggage accordingly. *Do not put essentials in your main case.*

If you are travelling by air, your suitcase may be inaccessible for hours.

So, have at the ready:

- Nappies and travel wipes.
- If you are bottle feeding, more formula than you think you will need.
- A change of clothes for the baby (and yourself, if you have room).
- Toys and books, which you don't mind losing, that can be handed out slowly, one at a time.
- If you are travelling for many hours, consider talking to your GP about taking a mild sedative for your baby.
- If you are flying, ask for a skycot when you book your seat, although not all flights have these.
- Have something for your baby to suck on, in case changes in air pressure give him earache.

Family-Friendly Tour Operators

These are tour operators who actively encourage families to travel with them.

Company	Baby/Child Facilities	Cost Reductions	Comments
Club Med (Tel: 0171 581 1161)	Babysitting and kids' clubs (3–5 and 6–11) in all resorts. Baby clubs at some destinations.	For under-12s: size of reduction depends on season.	Expensive. Do not be seduced by the brochure. Talk to someone who has been to Club Med to get a realistic picture.
Cosmos (Tel: 0161 480 5799)	Kids' club (3–9) but no babysitting.	Under-twos: £15. Children free at some resorts.	Good-value packages for European sunspots.

Company	Baby/Child Facilities	Cost Reductions	Comments
First choice (Tel: 0161 742 2228)	Kids' club (15 months+). Reps may arrange babysitting.	First child free or from £5 per child.	Good-value packages, especially for the USA.
Thompson Holidays (Tel: 0990 143503)	Toddlers' play area. Babysitting £5 per hour for children over two.	Under-twos are free.	Basic package holidays.
Sunworld (Tel: 0990 550440)	Creche facilities from six months. Babysitting is extra.	Under-twos: £15.	Basic packages for Europe.
Mark Warner (Tel: 0171 761 7000)	Kids' club for children over four months. Free listening service in the evening.	Under-twos: £60 per week.	Known primarily for their ski holidays although they have resorts across Europe. Sometimes perceived as a Club Med 'also ran'. Talk to someone who has been to the resort you are interested in.

What You Will Need When You Get There

If you are travelling in the UK and do not want to lug a bootload of baby gear, the Baby Equipment Hirers Association (Tel: 01831 310355, or if you have problems: 0113 278 5560) may be able to put you in touch with a local hirer who can organise equipment to be ready for you at your destination.

One parent told us that if they had to take one item on a beach holiday with their baby, it would be a small inflatable boat. Not only is it fun in the water but it can be used as a mini-playpen/baby lounger in the shade.

Even if equipment is provided, test it carefully before you put your baby in it. Don't risk your baby's life with rickety items – especially highchairs and cots.

If you're staying in a place where cots aren't provided you can buy or hire a travel cot (see pp. 199–201).

Sun and Sea Holidays

The Health Education Authority runs the Sun Know How Campaign which is designed to raise awareness of the need for protection in the sun. This is because sunburn during childhood or over-exposure to UV (ultraviolet) can lead to skin cancer years later.

The Sun Know How Campaign has linked up with a number of retailers to provide products that are designed and tested to give children protection even in tropical sun.

High street own-brand sun products following this code currently include Asda, Boots, BHS, Sainsbury's, Superdrug, Tesco and the Early Learning Centre and the numbers are growing. Look out for products carrying the HEA logo combined with a sun safety code presented in five circles or tags guaranteeing UV protection.

Sun Protection

- The best way to defend your baby against the harmful effects of the sun is to keep him out of it.
- If you don't want to stay inside you may need to resort to a parasol or canopy on his buggy in conjunction with a hat and protective clothing. You need the protective clothing because parasols are not designed to give total protection. Some are so flimsy that the light can shine straight through.
- You may also need an easily transportable shelter, like the Pod (see Product Table below) or a beach cabana.

Hats

- Ignore cute designs and go for either a wide-brim or a 'legionnaire' design with a peak at the front and a flap at the back (see Product Table below).
- It must stay on, so you may need one with ties or an elastic.

Clothes
- Be particularly wary about T-shirts. UV can get through a thin one and cause sunburn. A thin T-shirt offers minimal protection (around SPF 5) and a thicker one may feel so hot that your child will insist on stripping off. There are special lines of clothes designed to block the sun with an SPF of at least 30. Sun Know How fabrics are tested to ensure that they block at least 98% of UV (available from catalogue and some of the retailers listed on p. 144).

Sunscreen
- A child's skin is thinner than an adult's. And children don't produce as much melanin to protect the skin from harmful rays, so sunscreen is a must (see Product Table below).
- You need to buy sun creams formulated for children and babies, as adult creams may irritate their delicate skin.
- You can have either a chemical type that absorbs radiation but allows some rays to reach the skin, or a physical type containing particles that reflect the sun. These sometimes offer total protection but may be difficult to apply.
- SPF 15 is normally considered the minimum strength for children. Don't pay extra for creams offering SPFs over 30 as the protection does not increase that significantly.

Insect Repellent
- In Boots you will find Baby Soltan Insect Repellent Wipes (£2.99 for a pack of 25).

Swimwear
- For suppliers of swim nappies and bathing costumes, see Product Table below.
- It's best to buy two swim nappies so that one can dry while the other is in use.

Product Table

Products for Sun and Sea Holidays			
Product	**Price**	**Stockist**	**Comments**
Tents or Cabanas – lightweight folding tents offering sun protection.			
Note: If you like one that is not listed below, check that it guarantees proper protection before you buy it.			
Baby Cabana Big Cabana	£25.99 £49.99	Great Little Trading Company (Tel: 0990 673008)	Smaller one fits only babies or small children. Larger one will fit you as well. Both fold easily to fit into carry bag (supplied).
The Pod	£49.99	Daisy and Tom, Urchin, Protection Outdoors (Tel: 0131 555 1020)	Offers UV Protection Factor 40 to a gaggle of small children or an adult and baby. Packs away easily and weighs less than 1kg.
Sun Hats			
JoJo flap hats and sun hats for three months+	£9.99	JoJo (Mail order: 0171 351 4112)	Two good, shady designs to co-ordinate with swim nappies.
Reversible legionnaire hat and Beanie hat (broad brim) fits 0+	£5	Boots	These come in bold colours. The cheapest we could find in these designs.
The original flap hat for 0+	£10.99	Urchin (Tel: 01672 871515)	Tiny 'foreign legion' hat – swim nappy to match (£10.99).

Products for Sun and Sea Holidays (continued)

Product	Price	Stockist	Comments
'Sunproof' Swimwear and T-shirts – also look out for new lines in multiples (e.g. Boots) listed on p. 143.			
Swimwear, surfsuits, sunproof T-shirt and short sets	£13–£14	Boots	If your local branch is small, you can order these through the *Your Baby and You* magazine £1.50 (Spring/Summer 1999) from Boots stores.
Stingray		Stingray brochure (Tel: 01799 523323)	Not as extensive as Sun Know How but you may prefer their designs.
Sunscreens – there are many excellent products available. These three are chosen as an example of what is available across the country.			
Soltan Baby Protection SPF 50 Roll-on Lotion 👑	£4.99	Boots	The whole Soltan range is widely respected. Many mothers found this roll-on easy to apply and use. The necessarily small bottles make it last a relatively short time.
Ambre Solaire Sun Block Milk for Kids SPF 35	£10.99 for 200ml	Chemists	Water-resistant, reliable.
Uvistat Babysun Ultrablock Suncream SPF 30 ☺	£7.39 for 50g	Chemists	A traditional favourite.

Products for Sun and Sea Holidays (continued)

Product	Price	Stockist	Comments
Swim Nappies			
Floaties Aquanappies	£5.95	Tel: 01252 316626	Elasticated waist and leg-holes make them extremely effective but can be uncomfortable for chunkier babies.
Kooshies Swim Nappy ☺	£7.99	PHP (Tel: 0870 6070545) available by mail order or sold in many UK leisure centre shops.	Some people found tying the bow a fiddle but still hugely popular and – most important – very reliable.
JoJo swimming shorts/ nappies (have co-ordinating hat)	£9.99	JoJo (Mail order: 0171 351 4112)	Not tested – but extremely well-disguised swim nappies. Look like normal swimwear.

Learning to Swim

Float suits allow children to be buoyant in the water. If you want your baby to start swimming lessons relatively early, take advice from the swimming instructors at your local pool before buying these.

There are two types of float suits:

- Swimsuits with eight removable buoyancy floats. You remove the floats one by one as your child learns to swim. Boy and girl versions are available from JoJo (£31.99). Sizes: two to three years and four to five years.
- Swimsuits with two inflatable flotation pads. Boy and girl versions of Floaties Swim Mate are available (£19.99). Sizes: 12 to 24 months and two to four years. Buoyancy is altered by the amount of air in the pads.

JoJo also stock the extremely popular Floaties armbands (£4.99). Sizes: three to 24 months and two to five years. (It's very important to buy ones that fit well.) If you need a gimmick to make your baby wear these, duck armbands are available from Urchins (£4.50) as well as a duck swim ring (£3.90).

Fun in the Water
The much-loved Tomy Swimseat, which allows a small baby to bob up and down in a supporting floating seat (£9.50), is available in two sizes from Perfectly Happy People (PHP) mail order (Tel: 0870 6070545).

PHP can also supply a baby holiday pack (£9.95). This is a clear holdall containing a legionnaire-style hat and armbands. The bag is large enough to take a towel and sun cream as well. State the age/size of your baby when you order.

If your baby enjoys playing with Flexi Floats (the long foam 'sausages' available in many public swimming baths), you can buy them (at £4.99 each or £13.99 for three plus £1.50 p&p). Call Swim BG (Tel: 0800 220292) for details.

Section 2: Optional Extras

Baby Bouncers

A bouncer, used properly, will amuse your baby and exercise his leg muscles. A few babies loathe the bounce sensation (so keep your receipt) but most will happily bungee away for five to 10 minutes. A bouncer may keep your baby safely amused but you must never leave him in it unattended. These are suitable for babies of four months and over, who can support their own heads.

There are two main types of baby bouncer. There's the traditional type – a seat or harness on a long sprung chain or rope that you attach to a doorframe using a metal clamp. Or there's a free-standing model, with the harness suspended from a special metal frame.

Checklist
Doorframes

- If you are buying a traditional bouncer to suspend from your doorframe, check that the frames are suitable. They must be solid and absolutely straight. The architrave must be at least 2cm proud of the wall to allow the clamping mechanism to fit properly.
- Also check that the doorframes are identically fitted on either side of the door.

Sloping Floors and Doors

- If either the frame or the floor slopes, your baby will end up hopping on one leg.
- If the doorframes are inappropriate, buy a free-standing model.

Space

- If you have lots of space, the Tippitoes Trio (see Product Table opposite) is probably the safest option, as it has its

own frame to hang a bouncer on. But these do take up a lot of room both to use and to store.
- The really easy to use, wipe-clean models (e.g. the Mothercare Bird Bouncer) will take up far more room than the fabric versions (e.g. Mornbrook Baby Bouncer).

Older Siblings
- Consider whether the bouncer might turn your infant into a baby-baiting activity centre.

Ease of Use and Washability
- Ignore anything with poppers, or lots of buttons or straps, as it will be difficult to lift your baby in and out.
- Make sure that any clips, including the one attaching the seat to the harness, are easy to use. You will not be able to wrestle with them and hold a baby at the same time.
- The bouncer must be washable.

Comfort
- If it has a crossbar to fasten the harness to the long ropes, make sure that the bar is not so low that it hinders your baby's upward mobility.

Product Table

Baby Bouncers		
Brand and Price	**Stockists**	**Comments**
Mothercare Bird Bouncer £34.99 ♛	Mothercare	Easy to use; no fiddly assembly, wipes clean. Recommended for babies of five months+ (6–13kg).

Baby Bouncers (continued)

Brand and Price	Stockists	Comments
Mornbrook Baby Bouncer (£23)	Independent retailers and Littlewoods Home Shopping (Tel: 0345 888222)	Sturdy and fits securely to doorframe, although may prove tricky to lever baby in and out. Looks old-fashioned compared to model above but no complaints on fun value.
Tippitoes (£19.99) ☺	Tesco Direct (Tel: 0345 024024)	Well made; easy to get baby in and out; good support for waist and lower back. Minimal storage space required.
Tippitoes Trio (£37.99) ♛	As above and independent retailers, John Lewis	Baby bouncer (as above) comes with lightweight portable frame that can be used indoors or outside. You can also suspend a baby car seat from the frame or toys on special chains provided.

Baby Walkers

These have not been tested, as Liverpool Trading Standards Officers have several court cases pending against baby walker manufacturers.

The outcome of these cases could affect styles of baby walkers across the UK which would make this section out of date almost as soon as you have finished reading it.

Industry experts believe that most baby walker accidents occur when they are in use without parental supervision – for example, if a baby is using one on a landing and goes toppling down the stairs.

If you fancy buying one, treat it as a toy not a walking aid. Don't leave your baby in it for long periods and always make sure that he is supervised.

As well as stairs, never place the walker on the tops of tables, near unguarded tiles or sharp corners and knobs on furniture. Access to kitchen gadgets that the baby might pull down on himself while using the walker should also be avoided.

♛ An alternative is the 'stationary entertainer' like the Graco Fun Rock (£49.99). This looks like a walker but the baby can only bounce in a stationary position rather than walk around.

Baby Carriers

These are useful if you want to keep your baby close but your hands free. Whether strapped to your front or back, they can make trips to the supermarket easier and a walk with friends less hard work and more fun.

But oh, the pain, as from the backpack behind, little angel grabs your hair with his Pit Bull paws and won't let go . . . A front carrier or sling is less trouble but is only useful for the first months of your baby's life when his favoured method of testing your affection is to throw up on your new 'dry clean only' jacket.

Shopping List
- Front carrier/sling – for smaller babies.
- Back carrier – for babies who can support their heads and bodies (six months+).

Checklist
- A baby carrier is a good idea if you tend to visit places that are unsuitable for a buggy (e.g. crowded narrow streets, steep hills, and muddy lanes).
- They're also useful if you want to go out with another child using the buggy.
- If you want one for a one-week summer holiday – rent or buy one second-hand. They are expensive for short-term use.
- Baby carriers are *not* a good idea if you are a petite parent with a large, heavy baby, or have back problems.
- Don't be tempted to buy a complex back carrier for solitary walks – you will have problems heaving the back carrier on and off.

- Don't attempt to try these out with an eight-month bump. Delay the purchase until your baby has arrived.

Features to Suit You
- If both parents want to use the carrier, a non-sexist model is essential – no frills or flowers.
- A new mother's muscles will be soft, so it is essential not to put any additional strain on the back and shoulders. A good design will ensure that the load is evenly spread across the shoulders, waist and hips.
- The straps must be padded and easily adjustable – especially if different people are going to use the carrier.
- Carriers get dirty. If your baby is inclined to dribble it is essential to have a washable/spongeable model.

Features to Suit Your Baby
- The carrier should give good head and back support. Your baby should look and feel snug and secure.
- There also needs to be enough leg space. Ensure that the leg holes will accommodate chunky thighs encased in a snowsuit. For cold days, babies need to be well wrapped up.

Front Carriers
- Front carriers are particularly good if you use public transport with a small baby.
- They're also useful if you want to keep a new baby close while you do household chores. (But don't do anything involving hot food or drink.)
- If you are considering a pouch-type carrier that straps to your chest, it should be high enough for your baby's head to nestle against your breast bone.
- You should feel totally secure with your baby in the carrier. If you find that you need to support his head or body with your hands, the carrier is not doing its job. (The exception to this is if you are wearing a front carrier and need to lean sharply forward.)
- Some models can be used on both your front and your back. This flexibility may be important to some purchasers.

Back Carriers

- It may feel fine with an infant, but if you are buying a back carrier to last a couple of years, you need something that will still be bearable with a seriously bouncing babe on board. If your baby is very heavy, it is unrealistic to expect total comfort for either the schlepper or the schlepped.

Product Table

What we looked for:

- Safety.
- Ease of use.
- Comfort for carer.
- Comfort for baby.
- Ease of maintenance.

Front Carriers		
Model and Price	**Stockists**	**Comments**
BabyBjornBaby carrier (£44.90) For babies of one week to 10 months+ 👑	Most nursery stores, e.g. John Lewis, Babies 'R' Us, Mothercare	Although expensive, this fulfils all the requirements of a baby carrier as listed above. It attracts universal praise. 'Absolutely brilliant. Baby was contented and I could get on with the housework.'
Wilkinet Baby Carrier (£29.95 + £1.55 p&p) Showerproof cape available separately (£12.95, no p&p)	Mail order (Tel: 01239 841844) or John Lewis	This relies on your ability to tie knots. 'Far too fiddly,' thought those who gave up in despair. But this is a good-value carrier that can be worn in a variety of positions, including the back. You've read the book – you can get the instruction video (£3.50). Passionate aficionados were gushing in their praise. 'My personal all-time best buy,' said one. 'Lucy practically lived in it for months.'

New to the market this year is the Tomy Bellisimo (£40). This is probably worth a try if you can't find either of the others.

If you want a carrier that rests on your hip, the following are available by mail order (telephone for an explanatory leaflet):

- Huggababy (Tel/fax: 01600 890569).
- Slingeasy (Tel/fax: 01189 404942).

Back Carriers

Model, Price and Weight	Stockists	Comments
Bushbaby (£125) Weight: 2kg Raincover: £24 UV-resistant sun cover: £32 Buffer (pillow): £5 ♛	Mail order and local stockists: 0161 474 7097	For long-haul walkers with big wallets this is the one. The pricey extras are aimed at attracting the serious walker who will be out come rain or shine. There is a 25-litre storage compartment and clip-on stirrups to make the seat more comfortable for children with longer legs. Bulky to store.
TM GS-90 (£69) Weight: 2.5kg Raincover: £13 Sunshade: £5.50	John Lewis and independent retailers Tel: 01706 877648 for local stockists	A well-padded seat for serious walkers. This has a good-sized storage bag. The easy hip-loading system makes setting off a relatively hassle-free experience.
Bébé Confort Wheeled Baby Carrier (£68.60) Weight: 2kg	Independent retailers Tel: 01732 740880 for local stockists	This one is for Professor Branestawm fans. It's not only a back carrier but its retractable wheels allow you to pull it along when your back can take no more. It can also be used as a free-standing seat. It has an integral sun canopy. Perfect for a short walk to the pub for Sunday lunch. No safety harness included but you can attach your own.

Back Carriers (continued)

Model, Price and Weight	Stockists	Comments
TM GS-60 (£49) Weight: 2.2kg ☺	As for TM GS-90 above	Not as padded as its more expensive sister, the GS-90, this model shares the same hip-loading system. Probably the best value of all and extremely popular.
Tomy Dream Rider (£49.99) Weight: 1kg £	Mothercare, Daisy and Tom	Better for small babies. This is the lightest one we could find. It can prove quite fiddly loading the baby but once you are moving it is fine.

Baby Chairs

If you find that you are constantly carrying your baby and your hands are never free for anything else, you need a baby chair. These provide a safe place to dump your baby while you cook dinner or answer the door. Once your baby is around four months old, you may want to put up his baby gym (see p. 196) near the chair so that he can entertain himself for a while.

Bouncy chairs hold babies at an angle so that they can see what's going on around them. Their gentle bounce appeals to most babies and some carers like to put babies in one of these seats, rather than a highchair, for their first solid feeds. You may have to fight the temptation to leave your baby in the chair for longer than the 20 minutes or so suggested.

Shopping List
- Bouncy chair.
- Swinging chair.

Checklist
- There are two types of bouncy chair: a padded seat on a tubular frame that usually reclines, or a one-position angled seat on a wire frame.
- If you have bought a stage 1 car seat for your baby, and he seems happy enough sitting indoors in this, you may find that a bouncy chair is unnecessary.
- Also, if you are tight for space, a bouncy chair is one more thing to trip over and you'll have to store it afterwards if you are planning another child.
- If your floor is highly polished, you may find that the chair slides around.
- *Never* put one on a table. A fall could be serious.

Inclusive Headhuggers
- Some bouncy chairs include a headhugger in the price which is worth while for smaller babies but probably unnecessary for babies of three months and over.
- You can always use the headhugger from your baby's car seat.

Easy-to-Use Lap Harness
- You don't want to split your nails every time you use this chair, so do check that the harness is both simple and secure.

Fabric
- Ignore PVC-upholstered models. PVC will make your baby sweat in the summer and it is cold to the touch in the winter.
- Ideally, you want removable, machine-washable covers but in most cases, a sponge-down or a hand-wash is specified.
- Some people may feel that padding is an important component of these seats but many of the cheaper models offer good support with very little padding at all.

Special Features
- The more expensive models usually offer a number of reclining positions as well as more padding. Some also come with a play tray.
- The reclining option is good, should your baby fall asleep. You can lie him flat with minimal disturbance.

Product Table

What we looked for:
- Value for money.
- Ease of use and adjustment.
- Simple fastenings.

Bouncy Chairs

Product, Price, Age and Weight	Stockists	Comments
Chicco Swing Bouncing Chair (£26.49) Suitable from birth to nine months Weight: 2.16kg ☺	Argos; also available from numerous baby stores but not necessarily at this price	This chair has owners bubbling with enthusiasm. They think it's great value for a good solid seat. Particularly liked by people giving feeds to a baby in the seat, as it is easy to recline if he nods off. Covers are removable and spongeable.
Britax DayDreamer (£45) Suitable from birth to six months Weight: 4.5kg	Independent retailers	Heavier and more expensive than the Chicco, this chair has two advantages that you may or may not think worth £15 more – a clip-on tray and machine-washable covers.
Bettacare Bouncing Cradle (£14.49) Suitable from birth to six months Weight: 1.75kg £	Argos; also available from numerous baby stores but not necessarily at this price	If you just want a safe seat to park your baby in, this is the best value we could find. It includes a headhugger in the price making it appropriate for small babies. It has no padding and is on a thick wire frame.
Britax Cradle Seat Deluxe (£19.99) Suitable from birth to six months Weight: 1.3kg	Independent retailers	As above but nicely padded with a good bounce.

Swinging Chairs

These are a nightmare to assemble, madly expensive, are in use for nine months at the most, need batteries, take up far too much room but have attained godly status in some households. The reason: they can soothe most babies to sleep. As the manufacturer's PR puts it, 'You have a choice – either you put your baby in the back of the car and drive up and down the motorway – or you buy one of these and have the benefits of the M25 in your living room . . .'

These are an ideal second-hand purchase – put your order in at your local 'nearly new shop'. Always make sure it's in mint condition when you buy, and if you keep it in good nick, you can sell it back to them afterwards. (See pp. 8–12 for general advice on buying second-hand goods.)

Product Table

Swinging Chairs		
Model, Price and Age	Stockist	Comments
Four 'D' batteries are required to power each model (at a cost of £6). Manufacturer says this will give 200 hours of rocking.		
Graco Advantage 2 Swing (£69.99) Suitable from birth to nine months or 11kg ☺	Independent stores, John Lewis, Mothercare	Two-speed rocking and two-position adjustable backrest.
Graco Advantage 3 Musical Electric Swing (£89.99) Suitable from birth to 11kg ♛	Stockists as above	The extra £20 buys you a play tray, an additional rocking speed and music designed to 'lull your baby to sleep' (but which may well drive you potty). You can switch it off, although your baby may protest. 'I've had customers bring in a screaming baby, I put them in the swing and they are asleep in five minutes flat,' says a Liverpool retailer.

Books

One of the best gifts you can give your baby is a love of books. Well before your baby starts to read, he will appreciate the bright colours and simple shapes of picture books aimed at the earliest age groups. Later on, you might use them to stretch your child's imagination, to reinforce new words and concepts by asking plenty of questions and involving him in the story.

Shopping List		
Age	**Development**	**Books**
Around six months	Can hold and chew a book on his own.	Mini-board books Cloth books Books containing different textures or noises
Around 12 months	Can recognise a few words and may point at objects he's talking about.	Books containing images of objects and people that are familiar to him: babies, animals, food, etc Simple stories Books with flaps or pop-up books
Around 18 months	Uses single words. May be able to identify an object verbally.	Books with 'rhyme, rhythm and repetition' Stories with brightly coloured pictures and not too much text
Around two years old	May use two words together. Can identify parts of the body. Attempts to draw things around him.	Stories that involve situations he will recognise, e.g. going on holiday Stories on tape to listen to in the car or in bed

Young Book Trust is part of the educational charity, Book Trust, which promotes books and reading. For an annual fee of £36.50 you can become a member and receive publications, such as *100 Best Books*, a magazine three times a year and Book Week material. For more information write to: Young Book Trust, 45 East Hill, London SW18 2QZ. E-mail: booktrust@dial.pipex.com.

Young Book Trust has a new programme, sponsored by Sainsbury's, to encourage parents to share books with their babies. Contact your local library or health authority for details.

We asked Young Book Trust, the Children's Book Centre, Borders bookshops and Waterstone's to suggest their 'best buys'.

Waterstone's is dedicated to excellence in bookselling. Stores are located in nearly every major town. They not only carry a comprehensive selection of children's books but they also run a helpful mail order service, see p. 167.

We were stunned by the vastness of the Borders flagship store in London's West End and spent much more time there than our research genuinely warranted. The children's area is designed with stressed-out mothers in mind – plenty of room for pushchairs.

You are encouraged to read before you buy – in the café people were munching their croissants and noting down recipes from the latest cook books. When I visited the Ladies, I could hear pages turning in the next-door cubicle. Enough said . . .

Other Good Retailers
WH Smith has a comprehensive range of entertaining and educational books for both small babies and their older siblings. They are particularly strong on creative and interactive publications, e.g. sticker books to help learn numbers, letters, etc. They usually carry a good range of story tapes and most branches will happily order anything you want in either the book or audio department. First-time buggy wheelers will really appreciate their wide aisles.

Supermarkets, such as Sainsbury's, Tesco, Asda and Waitrose, often stock a small but really well-chosen range of story/activity books.

Book List

Recommended by	Title	Description
Around Six Months		
Young Book Trust	*My Farm* by Rod Campbell (Macmillan, £5.99)	Cloth book – animals and the farm Lift the flaps to reveal hiding baby animals
Young Book Trust	*Peek-a-Boo!* by Jan Ormerod (Bodley Head, £3.99)	Board book with flaps to lift Multicultural and interactive
Waterstone's	*Bouncy Lamb* (Ladybird, £5.99)	Padded cloth book
Waterstone's	*Pictures* (Ladybird First Focus, £2.99) *Animals* (Ladybird First Focus, £1.99)	Black and white cot book Babies' first board books
The Children's Book Centre	*First Disney Books* (Ladybird, £3.99)	Magic of Disney stimulates awareness of colours, first words and concepts
The Children's Book Centre	*Chug Chug* by Richard Powell (Tree House, £2.99)	Patterns, pictures and brilliant colours to fascinate babies
Around 12 Months		
Young Book Trust	*It's Bedtime* by Ant Parker (Campbell Books, £2.99)	Board book Bright and colourful pictures of a teddy bear, sleepsuit, etc
Young Book Trust	*Outdoors* (Frances Lincoln, £3.99)	Close-up photographs of familiar objects, bold and bright Subjects covering the garden, going out, holidays and toys
Young Book Trust	*Bathtime* (Campbell Books, £2.99)	Board book, multicultural Colourful photographs of babies playing in the bath
Waterstone's	*My Toys* by Sian Tucker (Orchard, £2.99)	Familiar everyday toys

Book List (continued)

Recommended by	Title	Description
The Children's Book Centre	*Tom and Pippo in the Garden* by Helen Oxenbury (Campbell Books, £2.99)	Delightful story about best friends
The Children's Book Centre	*Home* (Dorling Kindersley, £4.99)	Touch and feel book Illustrates familiar objects
Borders	*My First ABC* by Jane Bunting (Dorling Kindersley, £8.99)	Bold photographs of familiar objects Accessible introduction to help you and your child learn together
Borders	*Can't You Sleep, Little Bear?* by Martin Waddell (Walker Books, £4.99)	Warm and reassuring story Friendly illustrations, ideal for bedtime
Around 18 Months		
Young Book Trust	*All About You* by Catherine and Laurence Anholt (Mammoth, £3.99)	Multicultural book depicting children's feelings and family life Pictures of familiar objects with bold, clear text Encourages learning of first words
Young Book Trust, Borders	*Being Together* by Shirley Hughes (Walker Books, £2.99)	Humorous, interactive story Young boy and girl dancing, playing, laughing and reading
Young Book Trust	*Humpty Dumpty and Other Rhymes* by Iona Opie (Walker Books, £3.50)	Introduces children to the well-known nursery rhymes Ideal for reading aloud together
Waterstone's, Borders	*Wibbly Pig Likes Bananas* by Mick Inkpen (Hodder, £2.99)	One of a charming series of board books Appealing illustrations

Book List (continued)

Recommended by	Title	Description
Waterstone's	*Big Book of Nursery Rhymes* by Lucy Cousins (Macmillan, £9.99)	
Waterstone's	*Baby's Catalogue* by Allan Ahlberg (Puffin, £4.99)	Beautifully illustrated Catalogue of everyday objects for baby to recognise
The Children's Book Centre	*Noddy and the Birthday Present* by Enid Blyton (BBC Enterprises, £4.99)	Lift the flaps to follow Noddy's wonderful adventure
The Children's Book Centre	*Pingu* (BBC Enterprises, £4.99)	Colourful lift-the-flaps to reveal a hidden surprise on every page
The Children's Book Centre	*Little Mouse Goes on Holiday* (Tango Books, £7.99)	Pull-tabs and pop-ups reveal hidden animals waiting to be discovered
Around Two Years		
Young Book Trust, Waterstone's, Borders	*The Very Hungry Caterpillar* by Eric Carle (Hamish Hamilton, £4.99)	One of the most enduring and widely read picture books Visually exciting story of a caterpillar eating different foods
Young Book Trust	*Rosie's Walk* by Pat Hutchins (Bodley Head, £3.99)	A classic, re-edited as a board book Tale of hen going for walk, oblivious of danger lurking behind her but which the reader can see
Young Book Trust	*Pumpkin Soup* by Helen Cooper (Doubleday, £9.99)	Story about friendship and sharing Exquisite words and illustrations

Book List (continued)		
Recommended by	Title	Description
Waterstone's, The Children's Book Centre	*We're Going on a Bear Hunt* by Michael Rosen and Helen Oxenbury (Walker Books, £4.99)	A classic Beautifully produced, written and illustrated

Highly recommended by professional carers for babies from six months onwards are *Word Play Finger Play* and *More Word Play Finger Play*, two collections of Action Rhymes from The Pre-School Learning Alliance. These are unbelievable value at 60p each plus p&p. Mail order: 0181 684 9542 (credit cards accepted). For a catalogue listing all their publications, send an SAE to The Research and Information Department, National Centre, Pre-School Learning Alliance, 69 King's Cross Road, London WC1X 9LL.

Mail Order Books
Any of the books above can be ordered through the Waterstone's mail order service on: 01225 448595.

Two excellent children's book clubs are:

- The Red House (Tel: 01993 779090) which offers 'the best books at the best prices'. There is always an interesting selection for toddlers and pre-schoolers, and many of them are sold at a discount.
- For slightly older children, Letterbox Library (Tel: 0171 226 1633) specialises in multicultural and non-sexist children's books but you will have to look through each page carefully to work out which books suit your needs.

Letterbox Library supply a number of popular titles, such as *Farmer Duck*, in a dual-language format (i.e. the story is told in both English and another language – ideal for English children living abroad or children from overseas trying to get to grips with English). The 15 languages offered range from Arabic to Urdu (no French, German or Italian).

You can also order books on the Internet via www.amazon.com or www.waterstones.co.uk.

Books on Tape

If you want your children to belt up in the car, books on tape can have a miraculous silencing effect. They are also worth trying on babies who can't sleep. You can leave the room and they can listen to stories and songs performed by the experts.

The following tapes have been recommended by The Talking Bookshop who supply a vast selection of tapes by mail order (Tel: 0171 495 8799). They are also a good source of advice on what to buy – as they really know what sells.

- *Collins Nursery Collection* (£7.99).
- *Collins Lullabies* (£4.99).
- *I Want My Potty* by Tony Ross (Collins, £5.99).

You could also try Hodder Children's Audio (e.g. *Kipper Stories* by Mick Inkpen, £4.99) and *Storytime for One-Year-Olds* (Ladybird, £3.99).

Videos

Numerous mothers have said to us that, before their baby was born, they swore that they would *never* park a child of theirs in front of the video. Eighteen months on . . . they are at the front of the queue for the latest *Teletubby* tape.

Videos do have a useful place in your portfolio of child entertaining skills – they can keep your baby quietly amused for a few minutes while you attend to an urgent task. And some tapes, such as the *Barney* series, have real educational value.

Blockbuster, Britain's best-known video chain, recommend the following mixture of fun and instructive tapes and they stock them all:

The Blockbuster Top Ten
- *Teletubbies Messes and Muddles* (£9.99).
- *Banjo the Woodpile Cat* (£5.99).
- *Tom and Jerry's Bumper Collection* (£9.99).
- *Thomas the Tank Engine Spooks and Surprises* (£9.99).
- *Barney – Time for Counting* (£9.99).
- *Looney Tunes Bumper Edition Volume 8* (£9.99).
- *Teletubbies Nursery Rhymes* (£9.99).
- *Barney – Colours and Shapes* (£12.99).
- *Swan Princess – Mystery of the Enchanted Kingdom* (£12.99).
- *Paws* (£12.99).

During past summer holidays, Blockbuster have run an offer whereby, if you rent a video for yourself, you can borrow a child's video for free. At the time of going to press, they had not decided whether to continue this scheme but my fingers are crossed . . . (Shame on me . . .)

For details of your nearest Blockbuster store, call: 0345 413561.

Mail Order
Video Plus Direct stock over 17,000 titles, including children's favourites (Hotline: 01733 232800).

Multimedia

If you have a PC at home, your toddler will probably have already displayed a passion for the keyboard. Most of them are desperate to have a go. And both manufacturers and suppliers are making it increasingly easy to find appropriate equipment for really small children.

Time Computer Systems can supply a Learning Pack Plus Bundle for £99+ VAT. This includes Microsoft's Acti Mates PC pack. The mouse is a large Barney soft toy. Squeeze his hands or toes and he interacts with any of the *Barney* software also supplied for use on a PC.

Also in the pack is a comprehensive infant software bundle of six educational titles, a primary software bundle and a secondary software bundle. So if you fancy starting your little genius on GCSE physics, it is all there. Time sales line: 0800 771107.

Mail Order
The Great Little Trading Company do an excellent selection of educational software as well as a large stationary mouse for tiny hands, the Easy Ball (£26.99, including a popular children's CD ROM). This saves your own mouse from everlasting damage and allows your child to position the cursor with ease.

If your toddler has a real aptitude for computers, you will soon be able to progress from the *Jump Ahead* series (18 months +) to more sophisticated software.

For 24-hour orders call: 0990 673 008.

If you have access to the Internet look up http://www.babywow.com – a company specialising in software for 'infant stimulation and toddler education'.

For older children there is the Brainworks Club, a mail order company offering savings on shop prices. A catalogue of their CD ROMs is available on: 0990 143053.

Changing Bags

The changing bag is like a fertility symbol for new parents. It's as if we subconsciously think that tugging, lugging or tripping over these things proves our ability to procreate.

They really aren't essential for everyone. As one retailer put it, 'a bag is a bag is a bag – don't get carried away'. Their usefulness depends both on your own needs and your baby's feeding and excreting habits.

Some babies seem programmed to posset, poo or projectile vomit as soon as you attempt to leave the house. If you put together a full changing bag every night before you go to bed, it's one less thing your sleep-deprived brain will have to grapple with the next morning. But beware the bag and the baby. As you gently lower the heir into his buggy he may cunningly grab the strap and 'forget' how to let go for quite a while. Asphyxiation by changing bag is not a very dignified way to go.

If you don't have a changing bag, any old bag will do. If you want 'everything to match', buy a buggy that has a co-ordinating changing bag.

Shopping List
- Bags for short outings.
- Bags for day trips.
- Overnight bags.

Checklist
Unisex Design
- Fathers might balk at a pink flowery changing bag.

Shape
- It must fit into your buggy shopping tray.

Strength and Quality
- Your changing bag has to be really well made with sturdy fastenings so you can treat it disrespectfully.
- It also has to be fully washable.

Capacity
- If you are only going out for the odd afternoon a small bag is fine.

Internal Compartments
- You need one for dirty clothes, one for clean clothes and nappies, and one for bottles and food.
- What you want is always at the bottom of the bag so don't be swayed by lots of dinky compartments. In practice, they will drive you mad.

Detachable Changing Mat
- Even if you hate the changing bag, a small changing mat is useful to slip into your usual bag for days out with your baby.

Product Table

What we looked for:

- Rugged good looks.
- Good capacity.
- Easy access.
- Changing mat included.

Changing Bags

Model and Price	Stockists	Comments
Bags for an Afternoon Out		
Boots Afternoon Record Bag (£14) £	Boots	Inoffensive rectangular black shoulder bag. Includes changing mat, pockets and 'messy stuff' bag.

Changing Bags (continued)

Model and Price	Stockists	Comments
Mothercare Bottle and Accessory Bag (£7.99)	Mothercare shops and mail order	Holds four bottles or two plus changing mat and change of clothes. Navy floral print. Reasonable value.
Caboodle Changing Bag (£17.99) £	Independent nursery stores	All Caboodle bags are sturdy, well designed and great value.
Bags for a Day Out		
Great Little Trading Company Side Stroller Bag (£16.99)	Mail order: 0990 673008	Clever bag that is specially balanced to go onto the side of a stroller without unbalancing it. Can also be used as a rucksack. Ideal for travelling with a baby in a buggy as it's one less thing to carry.
Boots Black Rucksack (£28) ☺	Boots	Neo-Prada rucksack that is hugely popular for stylish design.
Nursery Emporium Nappy Bag (£260)	Mail order: 01249 811310	Yes, the price is right! This is a Bill Amberg bag made of calf leather with integral changing mat for high-flying design-conscious babes.
Baby List Changing Bag (£79)	0171 371 5145	Who would think such a chic bag could hold a pile of smelly old nappies! You would be hard-pressed to tell this 'designer' rucksack from the real thing. Exclusively imported from the US, you could use this as a bag in its own right, whether or not you have a baby in tow.

Changing Bags (continued)

Model and Price	Stockists	Comments
Overnight Bags		
Thiz Bag (£44.99) 👑	Mail order: 0700 780745	Although some users loathe the double zips which seem designed to snag on whatever old rag you've just tried to cram out of sight, many love the fabric and the removable 'end'. This gives you a choice of a large or small bag depending on the outing.
Argos Navy Rose (£8.99) £	Tel: 0870 600 1010	Comes with changing pad, soil pouch and shoulder strap. Sponge-clean vinyl.

Cycling with a Baby

If you want to introduce your baby to the joys of cycling, you almost need a seating plan to work out where to put him. Do you want him to sit in front of you or behind you, or trail along in splendid isolation attached to either your side or your back wheel? Whatever you choose, the experts are adamant about one thing: you will need to invest in proper kit.

Cyclists can meet with fatal accidents but the rate is decreasing. For instance, 1230 boys aged 15 and under were killed or seriously injured while cycling in 1985, but in 1996 this figure had dropped by over 50% to 552 (DoE figures). An increase in the number of children wearing correctly fitted helmets is considered a significant factor in these lowered rates.

As soon as a child can support his head, he should be able to wear a helmet. It is not advisable to take your baby cycling before then. If you are in an accident, the most severe injuries usually affect the head or face.

Shopping List
- Cycle helmet.
- And one of the following for children who can sit unaided (around 10 months to four years):
  — Front-mounted child seat.
  — Rear-mounted child seat.
  — Side car.
  — Trailer.

Wearing your baby in a sling while you cycle is not recommended, as stability may be a problem.

Helmet Checklist
Standards
- Any helmet you wear should preferably meet Snell B-95. If not, it must conform to ANSI.

Easy Strap Adjustment
- There is nothing that irritates a baby more than having his head fiddled with, but if the helmet is incorrectly fitted it cannot do its job. So make sure that the straps can be easily adjusted as he grows.

Comfort and Lightness
- If the helmet is not comfortable it will be very hard to encourage your child to wear it. Neither the pads inside nor the straps or buckles should irritate him.
- If it is light, it is more likely to be comfortable.

Fit
- The helmet must stay in place as you ride.

Child Seat Checklist
- Seats that fit directly onto the front or the back of the bike are the most popular way to transport children. These are suitable for a baby who can fully support himself at around 10 months and will last until your child is roughly four years old.
- Check that the seat has enclosed footrests with foot straps.
- There should be an adjustable harness.
- The seat and brackets must stay firm. If there is any movement while you are cycling, your stability could be detrimentally affected.
- Be warned that you may feel destabilised by these seats, particularly if you need to alter your usual cycling position.

Rear-Mounted Seats
- These seats fit over the back wheel.
- Check that there is good support for your child's head.

- If you have weight at the back you may need to balance your bike with weight at the front.
- Your bike may suffer from strain on its frame due to too much weight on the rear.

Front-Mounted Seats
- Your child sits on a seat in front of you while your arms go on either side of him to hold the handlebars. (These seats are not suitable for bikes with frame-mounted gear changers or bikes with drop handlebars.)
- These are not recommended for long journeys as they offer no head support to a sleeping child.
- If you think that your child could catch his feet in the spokes try a different model.

Other Options

In some cases, trailers may be suitable from six months onwards.

These resemble micro-caravans on two large wheels. They can usually accommodate two children. They offer total protection from the weather but you lack the close contact with your child offered by a child seat.

Before you buy:

- Realise that you will have to get used to towing it along and judging the extra width it requires.
- Check that your bike is in tip-top condition.
- You will need a crank length that is around the same length as your leg.
- Some people worry that trailers may not be clearly visible to motorists but a tall pennant and rear lighting should alleviate this.

Another option is a sidecar. These are similar to trailers but are pulled along next to the bike.

Product Table

Cycling with a Baby	
Model and Price	**Comments and Stockists**
Helmets	
Halfords Little Terra (£19.99)	Sizes: s/m (44–50cm) m/l (48–52cm)
Hamax Up to 3 (£19.99) Hamax Up to 4 (£19.99)	UK distributor: Fisher's Outdoor Leisure (Tel: 0181 805 3088 for stockists)
Trax Teddy (£12.99)	Sizes: s/m (43–48cm) and m/l (48–52cm)
Toddler Lifeguard (£14.99)	Sizes: s/m (45–48cm) and m/l (48–52 cm)
Giro (USA) Mini Moto (£24.99)	For infants: up to 50cm; UK Distributor: Madison Cycles plc (Tel: 0181 954 5421)
Rear-Mounted Seats	
Hamax Discovery 103 (£69.99) ☺	For children up to six years
Polisport Child Seat (£29.50)	For babies up to 22kg; available from Argos
Raleigh OK Baby Antares (£64.50)	For babies from six months to 22kg
Raleigh Cirius (£79.99)	Reclining seat – from age six months to 25kg
Rhode Gear Taxi (£69.99)	For babies up to 18kg; UK distributor: Madison Cycles plc (Tel: 0181 954 5421)
Rhode Gear Limo (£99.99) ♛	Crème de la crème – for babies up to 18kg
Front-Mounted Seats	
Hamax Discovery 101 (£39.95)	For babies able to sit up (nine months to 18 months)

Trailer Suppliers
- Burley – UK Trailer Company (Tel: 01208 815715).
- Cannondale (Tel: 0031 5415 89898).
- Koolstop – Neatwork (Tel: 01890 883456).

Child Seat Suppliers
- Rhode Gear – UK distributor: Madison Cycles plc (Tel: 0181 954 5421).
- Hamax – UK distributor: Fisher's Outdoor Leisure (Tel: 0181 805 3088).
- OK Baby – Raleigh (Tel: 0115 942 0202).

Nursery Furnishings

If you tell a shop assistant that you have come for the full nursery treatment, a gleam in the shape of a £ will come into her eye and you will find yourself buried alive in mountains of 'charming' bed linen, wallhangings and frilly nappyholders.

One sales lady told me how she delights in persuading mothers to buy a pram and highchair with co-ordinating nursery curtains, even though none of these items are ever seen together in the same room.

Shopping List
- New lighting:
  - Dimmer switch.
  - Battery-operated nursery lights.
  - Night light.
- Safer heating aids:
  - Room thermometer.
  - Thermostatic control valves for the radiator.
  - Thermostat-controlled fan heaters (not safe once your baby can move on his own).
  - Fireguard firmly fixed to the wall to cover gas, real fire or paraffin heaters.
- Child-friendly furniture – and children's furniture.
- Wallpapers, paint and soft furnishings.
- A parent-friendly chair for feeding, stories, etc.
- Storage:
  - For clothes.
  - For toys.
  - For nappies, creams, etc.

Checklist
Safety

- The question you need to keep asking yourself is 'How can a baby cause damage/hurt himself with this?' A

table light, for instance, could fall, shattering the bulb, leaving your baby at the mercy of broken glass and a dangerous 'live' filament.
- Once your baby is born, show the room to your health visitor. Her experienced eye may alert you to dangers you never knew existed. (For more on safety in the home, see pp. 228–41.)

Decorations and Safety
- It is essential to distinguish between decorations and safety devices. Safety items should look boring rather than inviting. 'Personality' socket guards and smoke detectors seem more likely to invite inspection rather than deter it.

Timing
- If you are going to decorate a room, do it well before your baby arrives, so that he is not exposed to any fumes or dust particles caused by the work.
- If you are stripping old paint be very careful. The Paintmakers Association says, 'even low blood lead levels can have detrimental effects on young children's intellectual development... medical advice is that children and pregnant women should not be near renovation work involving the disturbance of lead-based paint'. If you don't know whether the paint contains lead, you can buy a simple test kit from your local builder's merchant.

Demands of a Growing Child
- You need very little for new babies, especially those who spend their first few months sleeping in their parents' bedroom.
- But within a year your baby will be active – maybe walking around, pulling, chewing, climbing on anything to hand. So choose decorations that will be safe and sturdy.
- Ignore anything aimed at a particular age group – Teletubbies may be adored now, only to be despised later.

Your Own Requirements
- You will be using the nursery both day and night to dress, change and feed your baby so it must suit your needs.
- Do you really want to perch on a rocking horse for the 2am breastfeed, when you could have an armchair?

Essential Furniture
- Drawers or a waist-height cupboard are particularly useful if they double as a changing table.
- Children's wardrobes are a waste of money. If you buy a full-length wardrobe in the first place, you can use it to store toys as well as clothes.

Storage
- Toys and clothes have a fast-track breeding cycle that is difficult to suppress, so double the storage space you think you need.
- The following mail order companies supply storage units: McCord (Tel: 01793 435553), Lakeland (Tel: 01539 488100), and the Holding Company (Tel: 0171 610 9160).

Lighting and Electrical Needs for Nurseries
Lighting
Consistent use of brighter light for daytime and subdued lighting during the evening should help your baby settle into a sleeping pattern in keeping with the adult population.

Black-out blinds are sold by most curtain suppliers. If you are making curtains, you can sew black-out fabric into the lining but this does make curtains heavy.

Dimmer Switches
Fit this to your main light and you can alter the intensity of light in an instant. With a dimmer switch you should really have no need for a night light, as these perform the same task.

Night Lights
Many supposed 'night lights' are glorified table lamps complete with attendant risks. The safe choices are:

- Night lights that meet the standard BS EN 609582.10/1990 rev (*not* BS EN 609582.4/1990, as this is a standard for table lamps).
- A battery-powered light.
- A nursery monitor with an integral night light (see section on baby monitors, p. 90).

Sockets
A good number of well-placed sockets makes the room versatile. You can switch beds and cupboards round without worrying about trailing flexes. If your child will be in this room for many years, anticipate later requirements (e.g. sockets for his desk light, cassette player and maybe a computer).

Heating a Nursery
Babies are unable to regulate their own temperature. Concern is sometimes expressed over babies being kept too hot by a combination of too many clothes, covers and modern central heating. But babies must not be subjected to extreme cold either. Take advice from your community midwife on maintaining the correct temperature in your home. (For information on room thermometers, see p. 80–81.)

Thermostats
Putting a thermostatic control on your nursery radiator will allow you to alter the temperature of the room irrespective of how strongly you are heating the rest of the house.

Additional Heaters
If you need additional heat, have a heater that does not get hot to the touch, and has a thermostat to prevent overheating. A wall-mounted, oil-filled radiator is probably the safest option. Fan heaters are dangerous for babies who are mobile enough to stick fingers where they shouldn't.

Product Table

Children's Nursery Furniture	
Supplier	**Comments**
Simon Horne – top-of-the-range supplier to the stars (Tel: 0171 731 1279)	All items will adapt for adult use (e.g. changing unit becomes a chest, wardrobe becomes a TV display unit, and bookcase becomes a work station). Prices: £1500 for a Bateau Lit cot that becomes a bed, then a small sofa.
Mark Wilkinson (Tel: 01380 850004)	The kitchen king also makes the ultimate nursery furniture (£985 for a Goldilocks cot).
Dragon's of Walton Street (Tel: 0171 587 3795)	Hand-painted nursery furniture at high prices.
Ikea	Stock levels variable but, if you can find it, good-value nursery furniture (solid wood chairs from £5).
Billie Bond Designs (Mail order: 01245 360164)	Children's armchairs (£95) and sofas (£180). Known for their range of hand-stencilled wooden furniture.

Specialist Nursery Toys	
Supplier	**Comments**
The Doll's House Emporium (Tel: 01773 513773)	Superb catalogue of doll's house items.
Rocking Horses, Robert Mullis (Tel: 01793 813583) Victorian-Style Rocking Horses (Tel: 0181 367 0605) Rocking Sheep (Tel: 01678 521232)	The first two firms can restore old rocking horses as well as making new ones.

Co-ordinating Wallpapers and Fabrics

Brand and Ranges	Cost per Metre of Fabric	For Local Supplier, Samples or Catalogue Details, Telephone:
B&Q	Paper only	
Laura Ashley – Mother and Child	£12.95	0171 437 9760 (Regent Street, London branch if there isn't one in your local phone book).
Bundles	£19.50	0181 744 1440
Anna French – Ready Teddy Go and Harum Scarum ranges	£16.95–£18.95	0171 351 1126
Designers' Guild – Tiddlywinks, Hopscotch and Toybox ranges	£19	0171 351 5775
Dragons	£14.10–£21.15	0171 589 3795 or www.classicengland.co.uk/dragons.html.
Freemans catalogue		0800 7319731
Mamas and Papas	£29.95 for 3 metres	Popular range (e.g. Tall Story); ring for catalogue: 01484 438222.
Mothercare – ABC Patchwork, Animal Story, Ollie Bear, Beatrix Potter, Winnie-the-Pooh, Tweet Dreams	£9.99	All illustrated in newborn to toddler catalogue available from Mothercare stores.
Nursery Window	£23.50–£27.50	0171 581 3358: top-of-the-range nursery furnishings.
Osborne and Little – Scrapbook, Charades	£20.50–£23.50	0171 352 1456

Co-ordinating Wallpapers and Fabrics (continued)

Brand and Ranges	Cost per Metre of Fabric	For Local Supplier, Samples or Catalogue Details, Telephone:
Poppy	From £11.95	01642 790000: fun co-ordinates and accessories for nurseries.
Premiere Baby	£12.95 (Curtains £29.95)	01323 410470: cheerful, bright soft furnishings
Sainsbury's Homebase	Paper only	
Sanderson – Dick Bruna, Pat and Pat Interwall, Animal Story – Blendworth Options 'Picnic'	£17.04, £12.50–£16.50, £15.75, £15.50	01895 251288 (telephone for samples). Sample books available from Interior Design shops. Main showroom is at 112 Brompton Road, London SW3.

Wall Decorations

Product	Suppliers
Peel-on/Peel-off Decorations for Walls. For the fastest nursery decorations around go for Stikarounds, large self-adhesive nursery characters that can be stuck to almost any surface and easily removed afterwards. Clingsticks, their 'sister' product, can be used to brighten up children's bathrooms. £	Leisurebrands Ltd (Tel: 01225 461161).

Wall Decorations (continued)

Product	Suppliers
Stencils	Stencil Library (Tel: 01661 844844) has over 1000 nursery designs and equipment. Mail order catalogue £5, refundable against purchase. Stencil Store (Mail order: 01923 285577).
Print Blocks. Wood blocks cut into shapes that you dip in paint and 'stamp' on walls and fabrics.	English Stamp Company (Tel: 01929 439117) can make up a shape of your choice but also has ready-made stamps available (from £11.95 for a four-inch size). Also at John Lewis.
Soft Wall Hangings	Spottiswoode Trading (Tel: 01903 733123).

Toys

Baby's Law says: the less you pay for a toy, the more he'll like it. 'Despite all the time and money we've spent on selecting educational toys, her favourite bath toy is an empty plastic Coke bottle,' says one parent. Another points out, 'No matter how many you buy, he'll still only have one or two favourites.'

Heartbreakingly, it is these very objects that are designed to give pleasure that can be the source of serious accidents and even deaths. Even if you are scrupulously careful about avoiding toys with small parts, you have to watch your child continuously. Balloons, for instance, that staple of all birthday parties, have caused more suffocation deaths in the US than other toys with obviously hazardous components.

If you've got the nerve (and a lot of friends), you can stem a useless fluffy toy avalanche by following this parent's example: 'When people asked me which toy to buy, I asked if they would be kind enough to club together and get me a car seat instead.'

Before you buy much, visit your local toy library. There are over 1000 of these nationwide, with more opening all the time. A toy library works like a book library, although there may be a small charge for borrowing. Details of your local branch are available from the National Association of Toy and Leisure Libraries (Tel: 0171 387 9592).

Shopping List
One–Six Months

- Mobile.
- Mirror.
- A tape cassette machine.
- Rattles.
- Textured soft toys.

- Activity mats.
- Activity arches.
- Activity rings.

Six–12 Months
- Bath toys.
- Baby bouncers.
- Reactive toys.
- Balls.
- Toys to encourage movement.

12–18 Months
- Board/Rag books.
- Simple puzzles.
- Pushing/riding toys.
- Percussion instruments.

18 Months–Two Years
- Basic construction kits.
- Matching and sorting games.
- Basic garden toys.

Basic Safety Precautions
- Tidy toys away when not in use. This will minimise the risk of trips and falls.
- However much a toy is loved, if it's broken it must be thrown away.
- Use toys for the right age. Mobiles and activity centres must be removed from a baby's cot as soon as he has the strength to either climb on top of the activity centre or strangle himself with the mobile. If you give your baby toys that are too old for him, they could be equally dangerous.
- Keep seriously fluffy toys away from infants. Children under 12 months can choke on synthetic fur and hair.
- Always buy established brand toys for an appropriate age from a reputable shop. If you break this rule, be meticulous about checking for loose bits that could be swallowed, or sharp edges that could cut or maim.

Different Toys for Different Stages

This does not describe all aspects of development but is designed to show why a particular toy may be appropriate at a given stage. All babies develop at different rates in different ways. Toys that thrill some will upset others.

Age and Development	Appropriate Types of Toys
One Month	
Startled by loud noise Can detect light, shade and moving objects	Gentle, calming music Mobiles Toys that reflect light and change colour
One–Three Months	
Can move head while lying Watches own fingers and moving objects Looks at bright colours	*In addition to toys above:* A safety mirror Greetings cards that he can see but out of reach for chewing by accident
Three–Six Months	
Sits with support Holds objects put into hands without watching them Reaches for objects	Play mat Rattles and teethers Soft toys with different textures Activity arch – four months+ Baby gym – four months+
Six–Nine Months	
Explores environment by putting things in his mouth Can hold and explore objects for increasing periods of time	Toys that can be thrown, chewed and grasped by small fingers Bath toys Baby bouncers Toys that make a noise or 'react' (e.g. pressing a bell makes it ring)
Nine–12 Months	
Can sit up without support Memory develops and may look for toys that have fallen May be starting to crawl and move around unaided Can pick up small objects	Toys that encourage movement (e.g. a walker/push-along) Balls Toys that your baby can squeak or move

Age and Development	Appropriate Types of Toys
12–15 Months	
Understands a few words and recognises some objects May begin to fit objects together or take them apart Can pull self up and stand without support	Board/rag books Simple puzzles Shapes that can be posted into shaped holes in a box Pushing/riding toys Percussion instruments (pots and pans)
15–18 Months	
Builds towers and knocks them down Can draw short lines on paper Pushes large wheeled toys Can point out objects in books	Building bricks Chunky, non-toxic crayons and reams of paper Picture books
18–24 Months	
If walking, balance improves Can walk upstairs holding an adult's hand Can match two identical objects Co-ordination improves – can feed self with spoon	Pull-along toys on strings Matching and sorting games Garden toys aimed at younger age groups, e.g. a low, sturdy slide Basic construction kits that can be added to over time

Toys and Standards
The Kitemark
This is the certification mark of the British Standards Institute (BSI). It is an expensive standard to maintain, as manufacturers' quality-control systems are assessed at least twice a year. Few toys have this.

The Lion Mark
Developed by a trade body, the British Toy and Hobby Association (BTHA), this is a symbol of toy safety and quality used solely by members of this organisation. Members currently supply around 95% of Britain's toys.

British Association of Toy Retailers
This sign is found under the Lion Mark and confirms that the retailer is a member of the British Association of Toy Retailers and only sells toys that reach the Lion Mark safety standard.

Age Warning Symbol
This symbol is currently being introduced throughout Europe. It means that a toy is inappropriate for children under three, usually because it contains small parts that could hurt him.

CE Mark
This simply means that the toys are meant to be sold within the European Union. It is not a safety symbol.

Product Table

Not all toys please all children all the time. If your baby is distressed or bored put them away to use at a later date – or take them back.

Model and Price	Comments
Toys	
Mobiles	
Wimmer Ferguson Infant Stim-Mobile (£19.99) 👑	Because this is black and white, parents tend to ignore it in favour of a mobile that co-ordinates with the nursery decor. But from a child development viewpoint, this is the best tailored to infant capabilities. It may clash but it's the biz.
Tomy Sunshine Activity Mobile (£18.99) £	This is good value. It combines with an activity centre which you can use on its own once the mobile has been disconnected.
If you want a mobile in a particular colour scheme, Boots, the Early Learning Centre, Mamas and Papas, Mothercare and independent retailers all do numerous models. If you have two, position one over the nappy-changing area as a distraction.	

Toys (continued)

Model and Price	Comments
Musical Toys for Infants	
Playskool Musical Moonbeam (£16.99)	As it plays music, it shines patterns on the ceiling. It shuts off after five minutes.
Tomy Lullaby Dreamshow (£25)	Similar to model above but highly commended in 1998 'Best Toy' awards.
Fisher Price/Mattel Sleepytime Soother with remote control (£25)	Activity centre with lights, sounds of nature, and a remote control that allows you to turn on music without disturbing your baby.
Cot Activity Centres	
Early Learning Centre Musical Activity Centre (£13.99) £	Larger than most, with a range of activities including a tune that plays at the pull of a string. Excellent value. Apparently suitable for three months+.
Tomy Activity Play Centre (£11)	Doesn't attach to side of cot but still worth considering for travelling, as it has plenty of activities for babies of six months+.
Fisher Price Activity Centre (£13)	11 activities and five sounds designed to hold attention of babies of five months+.
If you happen to see the Matchbox Teddy Bear Activity Centre languishing on a shelf, he is very popular with babies and parents but hard to find.	
Play Mats – suitable from birth	
Boots Noah's Ark Playmat (£18)	Plenty to do – includes rag book and musical donkey; an ideal companion for visiting baby-unfriendly homes.
Gymini Tiny Love 3D Activity Gym and Mat (£27.75) ♛	Don't be put off by the bulk of this – it is an excellent first toy, with an enthusiastic following.

Toys (continued)

Model and Price	Comments
Wimmer Ferguson Discover and Go Playmat (£29.95)	'Research-proven design'. This has the advantage of being adaptable for use in the car and some babies might prefer using it there, as it could prove rather lumpy for a baby lying flat on it.

Rattles and Teethers – for babies of three months+

Boots Rainbow Brights	A variety of textures and rings for teething – e.g. Twinkle Twinkle Little Starfish (£7.50) and Terence Turtle (£7)
Mertens Wooden Teethers/Rattles (£4.95 at John Lewis) £	Should bring comfort where other teethers fail.
Skwish (£10.95 at Hill Toy Company, Mail order: 0870 607 1248, or good toy shops) 👑	Amazing architectural rattle, teether, etc, etc. 'For ages 6 months to 106 years.'

Soft Toys with Different Textures – babies of 0+

Boots Denzel Dino (£10) ☺	We received countless fan letters for Denzel.
Whoozit (£15.95 – large size – Hill Toy Company, Mail order: 0870 607 1248, John Lewis, independents) 👑	This is the trendiest toy in town. Amazingly, babies like it too.

Toys (continued)

Model and Price	Comments
K's Kids ranges (from £7.95+, at independent stores and John Lewis). We liked Sidney Snail (£9.95). £	K's Kids have not yet received the acclaim that they undoubtedly deserve. Well-designed toys come in their own carriers.
Mamas and Papas also do a good multi-textured toy range.	
Activity Arch/Play Gym – for babies of 0+	
Boots Farmyard Gym (£20)	Clever design extras (e.g. carrying handle, carry case and velcro for adjusting height of toys). But soft toys may not appeal so much to older babies.
Tyco Sesame Street Play Gym (£15 at independent stores) £	This model has been around for years. It is a good, simple design that can be easily stored and is hugely popular.
Galt Playnest and Gym (£39.99) ♛	Particularly liked by parents of multiples, as the large fabric-covered ring fits two small babies and provides both support and interest.
Bath Toys – there are lots of 99p ducks and boats around, which suit most babies fine. For bathers who need distracting...	
Bath Activity Mobile (£16.75 John Lewis; Hill Toy Company, Mail order as above; PHP, Mail order: 0171 677 1020).	Award-winning arch on suckers. You store it by 'sticking' it to the tiled wall and move it for use in the bath. Comes with detachable toys.
Mischief Bath Time Play Set (£6.95) £	A traditional selection of bath toys at a fair price.
Fisher Price Stay 'n' Play Bath Bar (£5.95)	A small bar on suckers that attaches to side of bath and provides relatively splash-free water play.

Toys (continued)

Model and Price	Comments
Puzzles	
Dress-me box puzzle (£9.95 at Hill Toy Company, Mail order as above).	Three-piece wooden bunny fits into bunny-shaped hole in lid of box. Stored inside are interchangeable clothes and bunny faces.
The Early Learning Centre have an excellent selection of puzzles (from £3.99 for a wooden four-piece Pooh to a wooden alphabet play tray for £4.99).	
Orchard Toys 'Big Bus' Puzzle (£6.50) from good toy shops or Orchard Toys catalogue (Tel: 0115 937 3547)	For older babies with a talent for jigsaws, this 15-piece puzzle is full of interest.
Musical Toys	
Little Tykes Tap-a-Tune range of instruments (from £9.75)	More basic musical instruments are available from £3.99 at the Early Learning Centre.
Vtech Baby's First Computer (£17.49 from Argos)	Laptop which introduces baby to early words and music with nursery rhymes.
Pushing/Riding Toys	
The Cosy Coupé (£30 from Little Tykes, Tel: 01628 524949) ☺	Britain's bestselling children's car. It's tough, sturdy and always popular.
Activity Walker (£19.99 from Chad Valley, Woolworths)	An activity centre that can be converted into a baby walker. A good-value sturdy version of this popular toy.

Toys (continued)

Model and Price	Comments
Push and Ride Coupé (£35.99, Little Tykes)	A parent pole allows you to push this little car. You can take the floor out for older children so that they can push themselves along.
Building Bricks	
Stack 'n' build blocks and bucket (£9+, Fisher Price)	A first set of bricks aimed at babies of six months+. Comes in a storage container.
Primo is infant Lego suitable for babies from six months. Duplo is baby Lego suitable for babies from 18 months – prices vary depending on size of box. Available at all good toy stores and selected kits sold mail order by the Early Learning Centre (Tel: 01793 831300).	
Matching and Sorting Games	
Chad Valley (made by Tolo toys) Musical Activity Shape Sorter (£12 at Woolworths)	Shapes to post and retrieve, with noises.
Tomy Hide 'N' Squeak Eggs (£5.99 from all good toy stores)	This is a box of six eggs. They each have a cheeping chick inside, as well as different-shaped bases to match holes in the box.

Other Toy Suggestions

- Pull-along toys on strings.
- Chunky crayons (e.g. Crayola or Early Learning Centre own brand).
- Garden toys for younger children.
- Ikea's 'Murmel' is a children's tent for £19.90. This is good value and can be attached to their play tunnel (£14.50).
- Argos stock an excellent selection of toys which they will deliver direct for £5. Larger items may be delivered free of charge.

Travel Cots

A travel cot is a traveller's version of a full-sized cot, not to be confused with a carrycot (see combos, p.126).

You only need to buy a travel cot if your baby regularly spends the day in another household (e.g. with a childminder or your parents) and a cot would be useful as a playpen for daytime naps; or if you frequently visit places where a reliable cot is not guaranteed. Look for BS EN 1466:1998 – carrycots/stands.

If you are only going to use a travel cot once or twice, it's cheaper to borrow, hire or buy one second-hand. Even if they fold away neatly, they are still heavy to lug around, so you must be sure it's worth it.

Shopping List
- Packaway cot.
- Folding cot.

Checklist
- Packaway cots fold neatly into a bag for easy transportation but may be tricky to erect. These are best for air, train and car travel.
- Folding cots are easy to fold flat but may not come with a travelling bag and may not fit into your car boot. They are ideal for storing in a cupboard or under a bed at your childminder's house should your baby need a nap. They can also be half the price of packaways.
- Check the dimensions of the cot when folded so that you will know that it will fit the area you have available for transportation/storage.

- If you want it to double as a playpen, you may prefer one with four (rather than two) mesh sides so that you can see in.
- Ensure that it's easy to clean.
- Avoid plastic-coated mattresses, as they can make your baby hot.
- Don't leave the shop without trying it out. If you can't collapse it and put it up easily – it's not for you.
- If you are buying second-hand, you must get a new mattress and it must be one that fits properly. (See pp. 8–12 for more on buying second-hand baby equipment.)

Product Table

What we looked for:

- Easy erection/dismantling.
- Spongeability/washable covers.
- Strength and stability when ready for use.

Travel Cots

Model and Price	Stockists	Comments
Packaway Cots		
Mothercare Pack 'n' Play (£79.99)	Mothercare	Well made; with a little practice, easy to use; wipe-clean, can double as a playpen.
Petite Star Travel Cot with Bassinet (£79.99) £	Tel: 01923 663355	Included in the price is a bassinet or high mattress which makes it ideal for a newborn or to use as a changing station. Check that you can fold it up easily.
Brevi Weekend Travel Cot (£79.95)	Stockists: 01630 638978	If you can't fold up the two models above, try this one. It should take the most buttery of fingers less than a minute.

Travel Cots (continued)

Model and Price	Stockists	Comments
Graco Travel-Lite Compact (£54.99) ☺	Stockists: 01753 714315	The bargain buy. Easy to use but not sure if all babies would find it madly comfortable for sleeping. Fine as a playpen.
Graco Rollabed (£79.99) ♛	Stockists: 01753 714315	Not only is this light and easy-folding but it also has wheels for pushing along when it is packed away.
Folding Cots		
Chicco Travel Cot (£75) ☺	Argos or 01623 750870	Absolutely great.
Brevi Oscar 100 (£49.95) £	Tel: 01630 638978	The bargain buy but quite small.

Section 3: Necessities for Older Babies

Baby Food and Feeding Accessories

Once that baby appears, the Great Race is on between you and other local mothers to produce the best-sleeping, fastest-drinking super-burper on the block. Even if you are ahead in all these categories, you should bow out of the competition when it comes to weaning. Ramming solid food into an undeveloped digestive system could cause problems that may dog your baby for life.

Shopping List
- Commercial baby foods.
- Equipment to purée fresh baby food.
- Storage containers for fresh puréed baby foods.

The vitamin and mineral content of processed food will never match that of fresh, home-cooked food, and the texture and taste is often very different. So if a baby is weaned predominantly on processed baby foods it may prove difficult to introduce him to fresh foods at a later date because he may reject the taste and texture. Commercial baby food should ideally be used in emergencies or for convenience when travelling or in other special circumstances.

Checklist
Go at Your Baby's Pace
- Anyone who patrols supermarket aisles will find countless jars of baby foods inscribed 'suitable for babies from three months . . .' but remember that the manufacturers are in the business of shifting vast quantities of baby food. The earlier you start weaning, the better for the big companies.

- Judge your own baby's needs according to how hungry he is. Four months may be quite early enough.

Consider the Cost Implications
- If you purée food yourself, you will make considerable savings. A 125g jar of puréed apple for one meal costs around 50p. A bag of six apples costing £1 makes enough purée for several weeks.
- If you are feeding your baby solely on commercial baby foods, you may find that you are spending around £3 a day (or £84 a month) by the time he is nine months old.
- Once your baby can tolerate complex dishes such as stews and risottos, you can purée your own food for him.
- If you want to freeze portions in sterile containers, use an ice cube tray or see the Product Table on p. 209.

Commercial Baby Foods
- Contents are listed in order of decreasing size so if a jar contained apples, water, then oats, there would be more apples than water, and more water than oats, but quite how much more is the manufacturer's secret.
- The general rule is: the fewer ingredients listed, the better the product.
- Organic baby foods, e.g. Boots Mother's Recipe and Baby Organix, use ingredients approved by the Soil Association as being fully organic.
- Beware of giving whole-milk products (e.g. yoghurts) to babies who are too young to tolerate cow's milk.

Mystery Ingredients Explained	
Calcium carbonate	Mineral salt used to neutralise the acidity in foods and preserve their colour.
Caseinate	Dried milk protein used to thicken and add bulk and texture to food.
Citric acid	A cheap way to stop foods going off. Foods vacuum-packed with nitrogen are a better alternative (although neither of these are a good idea for babies aged under 12 months).

Mystery Ingredients Explained (continued)

Demineralised whey	Adds texture and bulk.
E300	Vitamin C.
Hydrogenated vegetable fat	Increases calories in foods and stabilises other ingredients.
Lecithin	An egg yolk extract used as an emulsifier to mix fat and water. May suggest that the food contains hidden fats.
Maltodextrins	Cheap, sweet bulking agents with no nutritional value. (In their hydrolised form these are used for the gum on stamps and envelopes.)

Baby Rice

Most professionals will recommend that you start weaning your baby on baby rice. This is available from all retailers who supply baby food. It comes in a box and you mix it to an appetising consistency with the baby's milk. You shouldn't have to pay more than £1.45 for 100g. Ironically, the two organic versions that are readily available, Hipp and Boots Mother's Recipe, are cheaper (at £1.99 and £2.65 for 200g respectively).

Product Table

What we looked for:

- Pure ingredients with no suspect additives.
- Value for money.
- Foods that the babies enjoyed.

Note: The supermarket chains are constantly refining and improving their own-brand ranges of baby foods. As we are concerned that the names of ranges may change between now and publication, we have left them out. This is not in any way intended to denigrate own-brand products – it really is worth giving them a try.

Commercial Baby Food

Brand	Price
Boots Mother's Recipe (organic, four months+)	Pack of eight 125g jars for £4.56*
Heinz Pure Fruits	163g jar for 48p
Baby Organix (Stage 1 food preferred to Stage 2 for older babies)	100g jar for 59p
Hipp Organic	Pack of eight 190g jars for £5.68*
Beech-Nut	113g jar for 63p

*If ordered using Boots Mail Order (Tel: 0845 840 1000)

Making Your Own Baby Food
Equipment to Purée Baby Foods

- A hand blender, such as the Braun MR305 (£10.90 from Argos), is fine for most purées.
- You can buy a small food grinder (£7.99) from Tesco *Baby and Toddler Catalogue*, Tel: 0345 024024) if you need to purée food while on the go.
- If you don't want to use your food processor but fancy a miniature version, try the Tomy Mini-chef (£19.99 from Tesco *Baby and Toddler*, as above).

Storage Containers

- Ice cube trays are fine for storing portions for small babies. Freeze puréed food in the tray. Once frozen, put cubes into plastic bags in the freezer so that you can use the tray for the next batch.
- You should also start saving all those microwave-proof lidded plastic containers that you get at supermarkets (e.g. when you buy margarine or ice-cream) for larger portions. Or look out for the storage containers in the Product Table below.

Baby Food Storage Containers

Product and Price	Comments
Tommee Tippee Pots and Spoon (£3.19)	Three pots and a spoon for fridge storage.
Avent Babyfood Containers (£6.50)	Four small jars which can also be fitted onto an Avent breast pump to store milk. Being clear plastic is good – you can see what's in them. The lids really stay on and will withstand long use.
Mothercare (£5.95)	Multipack of three storage containers.
Boots (£3.29)	Two pots and a spoon.

Fruit Drinks

A government survey revealed that 86% of pre-school children drink fruit squash on a regular basis – half of these drinking as much as 1.5 litres a week. Because toddlers and babies have small stomachs, drinking sugary drinks means that they do not have room for more nutritious foods. Instead they are full of 'empty calories' which can have a detrimental effect on their health. 'Squash drinking syndrome', identified by a study at Southampton Hospital, can be recognised by symptoms including bad appetite, poor weight gain, bad behaviour at mealtimes and diarrhoea.

Avoid these squash drinks. Get your baby or toddler used to having water or milk instead.

This section on baby food was produced with help from child nutritionist and dietician Marianne Williams. Her practice is based in Somerset (Tel: 01460 242490 for consultations).

Bowls, Spoons and Cups

Once your baby starts feeding himself, you won't believe how much mess he makes with a small container of purée. Your hair (and his) will be stiff with the stuff. It will be liberally smeared on every conceivable surface and, in the middle of this carrot-spattered scenario, your baby will sit ruminating on one tiny mouthful, looking like the infant chairman of some global organisation.

'Put down newspaper and take cover,' suggests one parent of twins. A large bib and a PVC sheet on the floor under the highchair are two other useful stain preventers.

Shopping List
- Weaning spoons.
- Weaning bowl.
- Drinking cups.

Checklist
- All items (spoons, bowls and cups) must be dishwasher-proof.

Weaning Spoons
- Special weaning spoons have shallow heads and long handles. Their design makes it easier to shovel the first tastes of baby rice into your baby's mouth.
- Once your baby can feed himself, he will find it easier to use a stubbier spoon with a wider bowl.

Weaning Bowls
- Plastic bowls with high sides are the preferred container for baby foods.

Bowls, Spoons and Cups

- If your baby is feeding himself, a suction base will help keep the bowl anchored to the highchair tray.
- Stay-warm weaning bowls (for babies of six months and over) contain a special sealed compartment under the bowl which holds hot water to keep the food warm. These are not essential but may be useful for babies who take ages to eat and then spit food out because it is cold.

Cups

- If you have already bought a bottle that converts to a cup (sometimes called a feeding system) you do not need one of these. However, most parents buy one at some stage, just to get their baby used to drinking from different types of cup.
- The cup should be easy for your child to hold. Most toddlers like to grip two handles but some are happier with a smooth-sided beaker.
- The cup should have a capacity of at least 170ml.
- The lid should fit securely.
- If you are still sterilising feeding equipment, check that you can sterilise the cup in your steriliser or microwave. If you are no longer using a steriliser, put the cup in your dishwasher (if you have one) or use very hot water, detergent and a bottle brush to make sure it is cleaned thoroughly.
- If you are looking for a cup to travel with (i.e. you want to keep a drink prepared in your bag), look for a cup with a cover or a spill-resistant feature.

Product Table

What we looked for:

- Dishwasher-proof products.
- Value for money.
- Ease of use.

Weaning Spoons

Model	Price	Comments
Tommee Tippee Heat Sensor Weaning Spoons 👑	£2.49 for three	A bit of a gimmick but a lot of new parents felt reassured by these spoons. They change colour if the food is too hot. Especially liked by those who heat food in the microwave, as undetected 'hot spots' can occur.
Asda Baby Weaning Spoons £	£1.25 for four	The best bargain buy, with a sensible-sized bowl for a small mouth and a long handle for easy parental feeding.
Tommee Tippee Weaning Spoons	£1.75 for five	As above.
Heinz Baby Basics Weaning Spoons ☺	£2.29 for two	Really liked because of their rubbery texture. Parents felt that babies who were used to the soft feel of a teat on a bottle would find this the most user-friendly.

Weaning Bowls

Model and Price	Comments
Tommee Tippee Heat Sensor Weaning Bowl (£2.99) ☺	Red bowl goes yellow when food is too hot and comes with an airtight lid for easy storage. If you like the heat sensor spoons, this is the bowl for you.
Asda Baby Weaning Bowl and Spoon Set (£1.99) £	An excellent price, for good solid kit.

Weaning Bowls (continued)

Model and Price	Comments
Mam Baby Weaning Set (£3.59)	The glamour model. This has twin compartments which you may like. The handles are specially designed for easy use, but you may find them a bit too clever.
Heinz Baby Basics Weaning Bowl (£2.89)	Because this is larger than most and has non-slip pads it was greatly liked. Its size means that it will be in use for longer and is therefore a good buy.
Mothercare Teddy Weaning Bowl and Lid (£1.99)	Extremely sweet but lid not 100% easy to put on and take off.

Drinking Cups for Babies Aged Around Six Months+

Model and Price	Stockists	Comments
Tommee Tippee Kids on the Go Sip and Seal (£3.40)	Multiples and independent shops	Hugely popular, especially with mothers whose babies cannot suck from the valve-type design (see Anyway Up Cup below).
Anyway Up Cup (£3)	As above	Revolutionary cup featuring a valve in the spout which will only release liquid when sucked. Great for some but others lack the necessary suction power.
Avent Training Cup Set (£4)	As above	Bottle, training cup, with straw and spout adaptor. As this can be used as a bottle or a drinking cup, it is probably the most versatile product and ideal for babies who love their bottles.

Drinking Cups for Babies Aged Around Six Months+ (continued)

Model and Price	Stockists	Comments
Tommee Tippee First Drinking Cup (£1.79) ☺	Multiples and independent shops	Good value; secure lid.
Boots Trainer Mug (£1.49) £	Boots	The best value. The one to keep at home. No leak-proof lid for travelling.
Mam Twist 'n' Seal (£2.99)	Multiples and independents	You may dislike the lack of handles but it does have finger grips and a good travel lid.
TupperCare Sipper Tumbler (£7.50)	Independents	Travel lid cover, and choice of handles or beaker for baby to grip. Although well made, difficult to justify cost for an item that you are bound to lose. Ideal for totally organised, wealthy baby.
The First Years Tumblemates Spill-Proof Two-Handle Cup (£2.99) ♛	Great Little Trading Co. (Tel: 0990 673008)	Cannot be spilt due to valve in spout. Lid can be difficult to use and spout requires a good, hard suck which may frustrate some babies. However, valve is easy to remove. Little Cup Set (£7.99), with lids and spouts, is great for travellers.

Bibs

Once your baby has passed the liquid lunch stage, you will discover whether he treats his food like an impressionist, post-modernist or a disciple of Jack the Dripper. It is up to you to match the bib to the eating technique.

If you use cloth bibs you can never have too many as they always seem to be in the wash. Forget dinky little numbers – size matters. The larger they are, the more clothing they'll protect. Plastic bibs have a shelf so less falls on the floor.

You will see a lot of bibs for sale with velcro fastenings. Unless you are prepared to trade the convenience of velcro for constant bib-buying sprees, ignore these. Bib-averse babies take great delight in pulling them off and flinging them, dripping with food, at the nearest person (normally you). Also, velcro doesn't take kindly to constant washes in the machine and can end up choked with fluff and rather useless. Old-fashioned tie-ons, ones with elasticated collars or moulded plastic bibs are more likely to stay put.

Shopping List
- Infant bibs.
- Terry towel bibs *or*
- Moulded plastic (pelican) bibs *or*
- Overall-type bibs *or*
- Disposable bibs.

Product Table

Bibs	
Type	**Make, Stockists and Price**
Infants	
Small soft terry towelling bibs for babies on a liquid diet. You could use a muslin but you may find these more convenient.	Mothercare Bib Pack (£4.50 for three) Boots Newborn Bibs (£4.99 for five)
Droolers and Chokers	
Wipeable, moulded plastic with a trough to catch missed mouthfuls. Sometimes.	Baby Bjorn Soft Bibs for babies of three months+ (£4.99); six–30 months (£5.99), available at Daisy and Tom and through independent retailers; for local stockists, Tel: 0181 994 9469. Tommee Tippee Catch All Bib – six months+ (£1.75) from Boots and most nursery retailers. ☺
Throwers and Smearers	
Lightweight, wipe-clean fabric bibs that offer wide body coverage.	With sleeves: Great Little Trading Company Long-Sleeved Bib (£7.99) ☺ Boots Sleeved Bib (£3.75) Without sleeves: Great Little Trading Company Sleeveless Bib (£12.99 for three) Boots Tabard Bib (£4.25)
Travellers	
Disposables.	Boots Disposable Bibs Pack (£2.75 for 20)
Bib clips.	Clips that fit into your bag and convert an adult serviette into a bib, from Great Little Trading Company (£4.99)

Highchairs

With highchairs, first-time buyers usually have one overriding concern: is the seat padded enough to cradle their babies' precious little buttocks? Given that Mother Nature endows most babies with pretty well-upholstered bottoms, there are several more important issues. For instance, will the chair's cunningly designed feet trip you up? Will it self-demonstrate the foldaway option with your baby inside it? Will its turquoise bunny pattern clash with your minimalist colour scheme? And, most crucially, can you get your baby into it in the first place?

Shopping List
- Highchair/table-top chair/seat-mounted chair (Look for BS 5799:1986).
- Five-point harness.
- Insert cushion.

Checklist
- A highchair is a good example of a piece of kit that you should buy to suit yourself rather than your baby. *If space and finances are tight don't buy one at all* (instead, see portable table-top highchairs, p. 222).

Classic Problems
- These include chairs that collapse at the wrong moment and chairs that are difficult to adjust.
- Some chairs seem to attract bits of food to hidden corners.
- Others do not have sufficient restraints.

- Then there are chairs with trays that can graze a larger baby as they are fastened into place. And some have a ridge of PVC that pokes into the baby's calves.

Tray
- This should be large, with a deep rim to stop food being pushed overboard.
- It should also be easy to clean and adjust. Removable trays make for efficient cleaning.
- Some models allow you to alter the height of the tray as your baby grows.
- Wooden trays are more attractive but they tend to have a shallow rim and can be stained by wet cups and bowls.

Seat
- You need a large seat that will comfortably fit your baby through to toddlerhood.
- PVC is more practical than fabric as a chair covering.
- Some models offer insert cushions to provide extra support for small babies.

Harness
- If your preferred model does not have a five-point harness, check that it has 'D' rings with which you can secure your own harness.

Storage
- Think about where you are going to keep the chair. Do you want it to double as a play chair and table? Do you have room to leave it out all the time or will you store it in a cupboard?

Portability
- If you are going to carry the chair around, either from room to room or in and out of the car, check that you can do this easily.
- It must be quick and easy to fold away and not too heavy. You may feel a fool grappling with a highchair in the middle of Mothercare but you will have to do this three times a day once you get it home . . .

HIGHCHAIRS

Folding Highchairs
- These come on a wooden or metal frame, have a padded PVC seat and a tray that usually cannot be removed. They fold flat rather like a collapsed deckchair.
- Some models, when closed and propped against the wall, have a sneaky way of sliding open and tripping you as you walk past.
- Some folding chairs fold down into a small carrier for car travel.
- They are a good choice if you have a convenient broom cupboard to store them in when not in use.

Rigid/Fixed/Traditional/Cottage Highchairs
- You may have to assemble these yourself. They are good, solid items, which can look more like furniture than baby equipment.
- They should have a removable tray so that your baby can either eat in splendid isolation or be drawn up to the table to eat with the family.
- If space is not a problem and you want something to blend with traditional decor, this is probably for you.

Convertible/Cube Highchairs
- These can be used as a highchair or folded down to become a low table and chair.
- They may be bulky and heavy.
- The chair/table option may mean that this will be in use for several years longer than a highchair.

Folding High/Low Chairs
- This converts from a highchair to a low chair.
- Many models can also be folded away for travelling.

Portable/Table-Top Highchairs
As highchairs tend to cost between £40 and £80 and take up considerable space whether they are in use or stored away, you may prefer a cheaper, smaller option.

The Best Baby Buys Guide

Chairs that Attach to Dining Tables

- These are portable chairs (at around £30) that clamp onto your dining room table and take up minimal space.
- It is essential to go for a screw-on model. The suction models are not as reliable.
- *But . . . if your table is wobbly, or if the chair is not fixed securely, they are very dangerous.*

Mini-Highchairs/Booster Seats

- Another bargain buy (at around £25) is a mini highchair/booster seat.
- These need to be attached to a stable chair or they can be used on the floor.
- Booster seats are for older babies, making the transition from highchair to dining room chair, who need a little 'lift' in order to see what's on the table.
- For travelling, you can buy a fabric harness which secures your baby in an adult's chair. These have the advantage of folding down to a small package. At £12.99, they seem a great buy but some babies spend the whole time wriggling about in them.

Warning

- When using the highchair make sure that your baby is secure in a harness, otherwise he can fall out of the seat or slip down so his face becomes wedged between the tray and the seat – this can be fatal.
- Don't put the chair facing a table leg or wall. Some babies push against these, sending the chair flying backwards.

Product Table

What we looked for:

- Safety and comfort.
- Easy to clean.
- Easy to manipulate with one hand.
- Adjustable in seconds.
- Large enough to accommodate a growing child.
- Compliance with British Standard BS 5799:1986.

Highchairs

Brand	Model and Price	Stockists	Comments
Continenta	Cottage Highchair (£115)	Independent retailers	Well-made traditional style in beech wood; no harness but 'D' rings provided; removable tray.
Mothercare	Pine Folding Highchair (£55)	Tel: 01923 210210	Solid pine but light and easy to fold; good-size tray with high sides; integral crotch strap.
Britax	Picnic Highchair (£49.95)	Tel: 01264 386034	Easily folded into own sturdy bag; tray has high sides; wipe-clean seat; integral crotch strap with three-point harness.
East Coast	Cube Highchair (£59.95)	Mothercare	Made from natural wood; converts into low chair with own table; integral crotch strap.
Mamas and Papas ☺	Prima Pappa Multi-Positional (£120)	Tel: 01484 438222	Four reclining back positions; seven height positions; removable tray with two positions; footrest; on castors for easy pushing around kitchen.
Mamas and Papas £	Futura Multi-Positional (£69.95)	As above	Seven height positions; folds easily; removable tray with five adjustable positions.

Portable Highchairs

Brand	Model and Price	Stockists	Comments
Mothercare	Table-Mounted Seat (£25)	Tel: 01923 210210	Easy to assemble; sponge-clean seat; integral crotch strap; 'D' rings for extra harness.
Tommee Tippee ☺	Tota Portable Chair (£30)	Tel: 0500 979899	Screw on; washable seat; easy to assemble.
East Coast	Clip on Table Seat (£26)	Tel: 01692 403461	Easy to assemble; folds flat; sponge-clean fabric.
Safety First	Booster (£12.95)	Independent retailers	Dishwasher-proof (it folds flat like a dinner plate).
First Years	Three-in-1 Booster Seat (£25)	Tel: 0800 526820 or Great Little Trading Company (Tel: 0990 673008)	Combined highchair and booster seat; folds flat; removable tray.
Mothercare	Sit at Table Seat (£24.99)	Tel: 01923 210210	Four-position seat; integral harness; detachable feeding tray. Folds to briefcase size with carrying handles.
Great Little Trading Company	Safe Seat (£12.99)	Tel: 0990 673008	Strong velcro back panel to keep baby or toddler secure in chair; one size, adjustable; fits neatly in handbag or nappy bag; ideal for restaurant, shopping trolley, etc.
Tamsit	Chair Harness (£13.75)	John Lewis	In red or navy; fits most types of dining chairs – handy for holidays or shopping; fits into a handbag.

Highchair Toys

Brand	Model and Price	Stockists	Comments
Tomy	Baby Vision Activity Spiral (£5)	Tel: 01703 662600	Spinning activities; shiny rattle; squeaking rubber ball; spinning ball.
Fisher Price	Take Along Activity (£5.99)	Tel: 01628 500302	Two toys in one; spinning globe with beads; elephant teething ring with three beads.
Mamas and Papas	Drumming Soldier (£6.95)	Tel: 01484 438226	Limited activity but colourful and chunky plastic.
Early Learning Centre	Farmyard and Friends Spin and Wobble Rattle (£5.99)	Tel: 01793 831300	Brightly coloured; three smiling farm animals that spin and rattle.
Brevi	Baby Drive (£12.95)	Tel: 01630 638978	Dashboard with nine activities, including push buttons, clicking ignition, and wheel.
Boots	Stick-on Baby Telephone (£6)	Boots	Squeaky coloured numbers; rattle and spinning buttons; push-up ratchet.

Buying Second-Hand Highchairs

- A British highchair should conform to BS 5799.
- Look at the seat – it must be well upholstered with no splits in the fabric.
- Shake it a little – is it stable?
- Does it have a five-point harness – if not, check that it has the rings to attach a harness.
- Check that the release mechanism on the tray works smoothly.
- If it is a fold-up or convertible model, check that all mechanisms are in tip-top condition.

See pp. 8–12 for general advice on buying second-hand goods.

Potties and Toilet Training Aids

People seem to think that a baby's ability to wee in a potty reflects their intellectual excellence (especially if their baby has taken to the toilet before yours has). This view is a load of . . . well . . . rubbish. There is no lasting significance about the time it takes. If your child isn't dry by three and a half, see your doctor but don't let your child know that you are concerned. Everybody gets there in the end – even little boys, who insist that they are 'too busy' to learn about the joys of the smallest room.

If your child is resistant to the whole idea, try reading him a 'pro-potty' story. *I Want My Potty* by Tony Ross (£5.99, HarperCollins) is particularly good.

Potty training is easiest in the summer months when your baby is wearing fewer clothes. Buy leggings and trousers that you can whip off in an instant.

When it comes to choosing the right aids, it's very much a question of 'horses for courses' – or, in this case, 'potties for botties'.

Shopping List
- Potty *or*
- Seat 'adaptor' that fits over a standard toilet bowl.
- Portable toilet trainer.
- Trainer pants (plastic-coated pants or disposables).

Checklist
Making a Choice
- Once you have decided that your baby is ready for potty training, try to find a potty that you think will appeal to him. Best of all, let him choose one himself.

Potties and Toilet Training Aids

- If he seems interested in the toilet, use a seat that fits on top (see Toilet Seat 'Adaptors', below).

Stability
- The potty must be sturdy and stable – anything wobbly could put him off.

Splashguard
- A high splashguard at the front is particularly useful for boys.

Portability
- You don't want to drop a full potty. Check that it has a handle, grip area or slot that makes it easy to carry.

Novelty Potties
- Although amusing for the majority, some parents are concerned that a child who has a novelty potty at home may refuse to use other potties and loos when out.

Travelling with a Potty
- If you don't fancy wandering around with a potty under your arm or even a portable toilet trainer (which can prove pricey), consider a Toodle-Loo Foldaway Loo Seat (see Product Table below).

Toilet Seat 'Adaptors'
- These are ring-shaped inserts that fit on top of the toilet seat to adapt the adult-sized seat for smaller bottoms.

Trainer Pants
- Trainer pants get a mixed reception. Some people think that they are too much like nappies for a child to be motivated to ask for the toilet.
- You could always give a pack of disposables a try – especially if you have a special occasion coming up or a long journey without many opportunities to stop.

Product Table

Potties		
Model and Price	**Stockists**	**Comments**
Step by Step Toilet Trainer (£22.99) 👑	Great Little Trading Company	The Parker Knoll of potties – the high backrest and side handles make it secure and comfy. Later it can be removed for use on the toilet, and the base converts to a step for reaching the sink.
Baby Bjorn Splash Proof Potty (£8) 👑	Daisy and Tom and independent retailers	The best designed of the standard potties, this has a high rim and a ring of plastic at the base that the child stands on as he gets up, to stop the potty sticking to his skin and then falling over.
Ikea Potty (£1) £	Ikea	For £1 it's cheaper than a travel potty but may not be as comfy as some of the others.
Mothercare Potty (£4)	Mothercare	A good price for a well-designed basic potty.
Strata Musical Potty (£4.99)	Tesco Direct	Press a button for accompanying passing water music.
Toys 'R' Us Doggie Potty (£7.99)	Toys 'R' Us	This can convert into a chair and stool.
Spotty Potty (£14.99)	Urchin mail order (Tel: 01672 871515)	This designer potty 'knocks spots' off all others.
Curver Seat (£4.25) ☺	John Lewis and independent retailers	Highly recommended by many retailers, as it makes toddlers feel 'grown up'. It's comfy and it's cheap.

Potties (continued)

Model and Price	Stockists	Comments
Travel Potties		
Tommee Tippee Potette Portable Toilet Trainer (£6.19) Liners (10 for £2.49)	John Lewis and independent retailers	A travelling potty that folds out into a potty base supporting a disposable plastic liner. Not as stable as a potty, and you will have to dispose of the full liner. Suits those whose babies insist on a potty when out, if you have neither the inclination or space to carry one around.
Toodle-Loo Fold-away Loo Seat (£6.99)	Great Little Trading Company	A sturdy plastic seat that fits on top of a standard-sized toilet bowl but folds up to 25×15×10cm for travelling.

Safety Gadgets

Home is a Garden of Eden for curious babies, full of temptations that could lead to disaster. Hospital casualty departments deal with incidents ranging from pots of boiling water scalding a curious toddler through to electrocution and poisoning. To prevent accidents, you need to be aware of dangers and take precautions where possible.

However, even if you buy every gadget available, you still have to watch your baby constantly. You will also need to teach him how to avoid danger, otherwise going into non-child-friendly environments – whether it be other homes or public places – could prove a frightening ordeal.

If you want someone to choose and install safety gadgets on your behalf, Little Angels provide a baby-proofing service based in London. Tel: 0171 581 1605 for details (mobile: 0850979022).

Save a Baby's Life
The Royal Life Saving Society UK is a registered charity that runs free two-hour training sessions entitled 'Save a Baby's Life'. This provides hands-on tuition, including recognising warning signs, techniques to relieve choking, rescue breathing and cardiopulmonary resuscitation.

For details contact: RLSS UK, River House, Broom, Warwickshire, B50 4HN (Tel: 01789 773994; Fax: 01789 773995. E-mail: mail@rlss.org.uk). For a free copy of the *Save a Baby's Life Emergency Guidance* leaflet, send an sae marked 'SABL' to the above address.

Shopping List
- Childproof locks.
- Corner protectors.
- Door stops or slam proofers.

Safety Gadgets

- Fire extinguisher/fire blanket.
- Mains outlet covers.
- Smoke detectors.
- Stair gates (see pp. 237–41).
- Stove guard.
- Window safety locks.

Checklist – Danger Spots Common to all Rooms
Doors

- Doors can trap fingers; or shut a curious baby out of the room, or out of the house; or a toddler may lock himself into a bathroom if a sliding lock or key is positioned low enough.
- If you have sliding locks on your bathroom doors, remount them high up, away from curious toddlers.
- Remove keys from locks.
- Consider buying door stops and slam proofers (see Product Table, p. 235).

Electrical Outlets

- A child can be killed or injured by sticking a sharp metal object into a plug socket. Fit socket plugs or covers (see Product Table, p. 235).
- Keep dangling light flexes well away from inquisitive hands.
- Fit additional sockets rather than having forests of extension cords.
- Do not buy 'character' night light plugs. These are an invitation to a crawling baby to start playing with the electricity socket.
- If your wiring is more than 15 years old ask your electrician about installing Residual Current Devices (RCDs). These ensure that your system is safe.

Fires

- Fit fire guards.
- Keep matches out of reach.

Glass

- Low panes of glass in doors or French windows can cause bad injuries. So you need to have safety glass. This is marked with the kitemark or the letters BS 6206.
- There are two sorts: toughened glass, which breaks into small blunt shapes on impact instead of shards; and laminated glass, which may craze but will not crack as it contains a layer of strong material called PVB. For further information call the Laminated Glass Information Centre (Tel: 0171 499 1720).
- Clear safety film that sticks onto glass is sold by retailers such as Mothercare. The best kits include tools to apply film. Put paper stickers on panes of glass so that they are visible. Do not use plastic stickers. Masochistic infants may try to eat them, and choke in the process.

Windows

- Fit window bars if your child could fall out.
- Fit window locks that allow you to let air in without your child falling out. But make sure that the key is easily to hand, should you need to get out in an emergency.
- Do not put any furniture (e.g. toy chests and chairs) near windows, as this may tempt a toddler to climb up and out.

Rugs

- Remove rugs or tape them down securely so no one can trip on the corners.

Tables

- Fit corner cushions on sharp corners (see Product Table, p. 235).
- Glass tables are a particular hazard. Ensure that they are made of safety glass, or replace with wooden ones.
- Keep tables uncluttered. Clutter is fascinating and delicious to toddlers.
- Remove table cloths. One tug could cause mayhem.

Stairs
- You can stop children putting their arms through banisters by covering them with a rail net (see Product Table, p. 234).
- For information on stair gates, see pp. 237–241.

Checklist – Kitchen Danger Spots
Electrical Appliances
- Ensure that flexes are not long enough to dangle off surfaces.
- Where possible, replace with curly ones or buy flex-free kettles and other appliances.

Cupboard Doors
- Buy child-resistant catches for cupboard doors (see Product Table, p. 235).

Oven Doors
- If your oven door gets very hot, buy an oven guard.

Hob
- A cooker guard will stop children being able to pull hot pans off the hob (see Product Table, p. 236).

Safe Habits
Many kitchen accidents can be avoided by teaching yourself the following safe habits:

- Use back rings of hob and turn pan handles away from the front of the cooker.
- Boil only the amount of water you need.
- Do not have a hot drink while holding a baby.
- Do not store knives in a block; keep them in a child-proof drawer.
- Buy detergents in child-proof bottles and keep them in a locked cupboard.
- Deter your child from climbing onto kitchen worktops. Magimix blades, blenders and toasters all pose risks.
- Do not store tempting titbits above the hob or anywhere that might encourage your child to scale the worktop.

- Load the dishwasher with sharp blades pointing downwards.

Checklist – Bathroom Danger Spots
Water Temperature
- Scalding water should be prevented. You can buy an inflatable tap cover for a very hot tap (see Product Table, p. 234) but it is safer and more of a saving to turn the thermostat down to 54°C on your hot water system.
- Train yourself to run the cold water first and then slowly add hot, mixing the water well, until the bath is the correct temperature.

Bath
- *Never* leave a baby alone in the bath – even if he is in a bath support. These are designed to help you wash him, *not* to save his life.
- For more on baths, see pp. 29–33.

Toilet
- For babies fascinated by drinking water or playing with water in the toilet, you can buy a toilet lock but these tend to cause so much irritation and embarrassment to other people in the house that you may prefer to go without (see Product Table, p. 234).

Electrical Appliances
- Do not keep electrical appliances (such as radios and hair-dryers) in the bathroom. If they fell into the bath when your baby was in it, he would be electrocuted.

Medicine Cabinet
- For information on these, see pp. 86–88.

Cleaning Fluids
- Keep these in cupboards with child-proof locks (see Product Table, p. 235).

Checklist – Garden Danger Spots

Gates and Fences

- These must be kept secure and well maintained to stop children wandering out or hurting themselves on a damaged stake or loose wire.

Ponds and Pools

- Water just a few inches deep can be enough to drown a child. (Rain collected in a sand pit cover has been enough to cause a fatality.)
- Cover ponds with chicken wire that is securely weighted down at the sides.
- Empty paddling pools, except when being used under supervision.

Tools and Sprays

- You will need a secure lock on your garden shed to keep tools and chemicals secure.
- Do not mix chemicals in soft drinks bottles.

Greenhouse Glass

- Ensure that your greenhouse is made of safety glass.
- Don't place garden toys near the greenhouse.

Garden Toys

- Ensure that swings, slides, etc are installed according to instructions.
- Situate them away from paved areas but remember that the ground can become rock hard in winter so bark chippings or rubber matting should be laid to break any falls.
- Teach your toddler not to push or pull other children on this equipment and not to run in front of swings that are being used.

Pet Faeces

- Parasites found in dog faeces can cause infections which, in the most severe cases, result in blindness. Thorough poop scooping is essential.
- Worm your pets regularly. Your vet can give guidance.

Toxic Plants
- Even daffodils eaten in large enough quantities are toxic. But there are numerous flowers, berries and hedging plants that are far more dangerous. If you suspect your child has eaten a plant and is exhibiting worrying symptoms, seek immediate medical attention and be sure to take an identifiable sample of the plant with you.
- Major garden centres tend to label problem plants.

Outdoor Vents
- If you have an outdoor boiler vent it must be protected with a large metal cage.

Product Table

Safety Gadgets		
Product and Price	**Stockists**	**Comments**
Banisters		
Safety First Railnet Deck and Balcony Guard (£19.99)	Tesco Direct (Tel: 0345 024024)	Weatherproof polyester mesh netting to fit on balconies and stair railings.
Bathrooms		
Kinder-Gard Anti-Scald Bath Thermometer	Independent retailers	Plastic card using liquid crystals to measure temperature.
Boots Multi-Purpose Lock (£1.99)	Boots	Prevents children opening toilets, washing machines and other appliances.
Inflatable Tap Covers (£2.95)	Independent retailers and mail order from Premiere Baby Direct (Tel: 01323 410470)	
Larger Inflatable Tap Cover (£6.99)	Urchins catalogue (Tel: 01672 871515)	This doubles as a headrest.

Safety Gadgets (continued)

Product and Price	Stockists	Comments
Electrical Sockets		
Safety First Socket Inserts (£1.95 for four)	Mothercare, John Lewis, Boots and independent retailers	Three-pin plastic inserts to shield sockets.
Mothercare Socket Inserts (£3.95 for 12)		
Doors		
Slam Proofers	Good nursery retailers	Neat U-shaped stoppers that fit on the door.
Door/Cabinet Locks		
Safety-First Cupboard Catches (£1.95 for three or £3.99 for five)	John Lewis and independent retailers	White plastic catch allowing door to be opened only a few centimetres unless opened by an adult.
Safety First Cabinet Slide Locks (£2.50 for two)	Mothercare and independent retailers	
Edge Cushions		
The First Years Corner Cushions (£1.25 for four)	John Lewis and independent retailers	Adhesive, transparent pads for sharp corners on furniture.
Fire Guards		
Hago Extending Fireguard (from £18.60)	John Lewis and independent retailers	Width: 107–152cm. Suitable for most gas, electric and open fires. Comes with security fittings.
Kitchen Safety		
Safety First Fridge/Freezer Lock (£1.95)	Tesco Direct (Tel: 0345 024024)	Plastic strap buckles onto adhesive-backed locks for fridges, microwave ovens, washing machines, etc.

Safety Gadgets (continued)

Product and Price	Stockists	Comments
Safety First Oven Top Guard (£9.99)	As above	Clear plastic guard prevents saucepans being pulled over. Adjustable size.
Medical/Safety Kits		
ABC Child First Aid Kit (£24.99)	Independent retailers	
Childminder First Aid Kit (£31.99)	Great Little Trading Company	See p. 86.
Safety Harnesses		
Clippasafe Harness	Toys 'R' Us and Mothercare	Adjusts to fit around shoulders and waist. Zips up at the back. Side straps can be used for highchairs. Straps can be lengthened for walking rein.
KinderGard Child Walk-a-Long Restraint	Toys 'R' Us and Mothercare	Colourful, elastic wrist strap between toddler and adult.
Smoke Alarms		
Universal Electronic Child Locator Beacon and Smoke Detector	Good hardware stores	Ceiling detector with wall-mounted alarm and red light that flashes in window. Battery-operated.
Video Guards		
Video Visor VCR Lock (£2.99)	Tesco Direct, as above	See-through shield that fits over the front of the VCR. Plastic cover to prevent little fingers and objects being inserted.
Window Safety		
Boots Window Lock (£4)	Boots	Fixes window closed or limits opening. Cannot be used with double-glazed or metal-framed windows.

Gates and Barriers

Don't wait for an accident to happen. As soon as your baby looks as if he is about to crawl, you should consider installing a gate or barrier. If he can get up the stairs, he can also fall down them.

Falls are the commonest accidents in the home, with falls down stairs often producing the severest injuries. But a badly fitted, open gate is an invitation to the Accident and Emergency Department, so treat these 'safety' devices with respect and caution.

Shopping List
- Fixed barriers to block dangerous areas from toddlers.
- Opening gates for doorways and stairways.
- Walk-through gates.

Checklist
Types of Gate
- A fixed barrier is either screwed into the wall or has suction cups to hold it in place. You cannot open it to walk through.
- A full-width opening gate has to be screwed into the wall. (The whole gate opens.)
- A walk-through gate has a doorway in the middle of a rigid frame. It may have a bar across the bottom which could cause you to trip. You often have a choice between a screw or suction cup fitting.
- Some gates come in both wood and white metal finish. Consider which will go best with your decor, as it will probably be a feature for quite a while.
- Look for BS 4125:1991.

Where the Gate will Go
- Measure the width of the doorway or opening where you plan to have the gate. The Child Accident Prevention Trust recommends their use at the top and bottom of stairs.
- If you want a model that you can move around, you need one that comes with extra wall cups or fixtures.

Fittings
- Screw fixtures leave holes in the wall but are more likely to be 100% secure. If walls are plasterboard, check for battening behind.
- Suction cup fittings shouldn't leave marks but may not be quite as secure as screw fixtures.

Opening Mechanism
- Can you open the gate easily from both sides?
- Does it open both ways – in and out?
- Is the opening mechanism child-proof but simple and smooth for an adult?
- If the opening mechanism is halfway down the gate it may prove tricky, especially if you are carrying a child.

Installing Your Gate
- Follow the manufacturer's guidelines. This is essential to ensure that you are using the gate as safely as possible.
- You need a friend – fixing a gate is a two-person job.
- Position any latch away from the child.
- Never leave more than 5cm between the floor and the gate's base. A large gap could encourage a child to try and squeeze through.
- A gate shouldn't be fixed too close to the back of the first step – kids can use the stair to help them climb over.
- You may find that you need to use longer screws than those supplied by the retailers. A power drill is the tool of choice.

Once Your Gate is in Use
- Do not let your child play on the landing or near the gate without proper supervision. He may use toys as steps to vault over it.

- Always close it behind you.
- Train yourself never to vault the gate. If you do this while carrying a baby you are putting both of you at risk. It might also inspire your toddler to mimic you – with tragic results.
- Stop using a gate as soon as your baby's head and shoulders are higher than the gate itself. He will probably be about two.

Product Table

Stair Gates			
Model and Size	Price	Stockists	Comments
Bettacare Swing Shut Gate 72cm high × 75cm–85cm wide (extends to 95cm)	£24.99–£27	John Lewis, Early Learning Centre, independent retailers, and Mothercare	This closes behind you, thus lessening chances of baby falling downstairs through an accidentally open gate. If carrying a load you do not have to struggle to close the gate after you. And it has an easy child-proof opening mechanism. Wall cups are required for fitting.
Kiddiguard Safety Gate 73cm high Fits all openings up to 130cm ♛	£49.99	Great Little Trading Company (Mail order 0990 673008)	An amazing 'roller-blind' gate that disappears into a 10cm wide holder when not in use. This is ideal for the top of the stairs, as it has no bottom bar. Has an easy opening mechanism and requires permanent fixing.

Stair Gates (continued)

Model and Size	Price	Stockists	Comments
Tomy Soft Walk-through Gate. Adjusts to fit openings between 69cm and 94cm £	£21.99–£25	As above	Folds into travelling case when not in use. Pressure-mounted and made of strong nylon mesh with padded edges on steel tube construction.
Mothercare Wooden Baby Gate 73cm high (extends from 70cm–99cm)	£24.99	Mothercare and Mothercare mail order (Tel: 01923 204365)	No bar at the bottom, thus posing minimal tripping hazard. But the opening mechanism halfway down is tricky.
Lindam Extending Wooden Gate 80cm high (extends from 65cm–103cm)	£24.50	John Lewis and independent retailers	Same as product above, only larger. Extensions available to order (108cm–156cm).
Lindam Two-Way Alarm Gate 75cm–85cm wide	£28.50	John Lewis	Alarm sounds if gate is left open. Extensions available.

Stair Gates (continued)

Model and Size	Price	Stockists	Comments
BabyDan Multi-Dan Gate 72cm high (extends from 62cm–109cm) ☺	£19.75	As above	No bar at bottom. Wall cups required for fitting.

Shoes

Shoes are only appropriate for babies who can walk properly. Until then, padded elasticated bootees are fine.

Buying Children's Shoes
- Go to a reputable children's shoe shop where they have trained staff to fit the shoes properly.
- Go in the afternoon, as feet tend to swell during the day.
- Expect to pay around £30 a pair unless you can find Clark's shoes as they pride themselves on a range of shoes in all fittings from £18.
- Once your child is mobile, his feet will need to be measured around once every three months.

Checklist
- Check that the shoe gives good support for the base of the foot.
- It must also support the heel firmly.
- Pinch the middle of the back of the shoe between your finger and thumb and move the leather towards the centre of the shoe. Go for the design that offers the most resistance to this.
- Look for a sole that will grip the ground, rather than cause your baby to slip around.
- The foot must not slip backwards or forwards in the shoe – check this when your child is standing or walking.
- If you cannot take your child to the shoe shop, some podriatrists suggest drawing round each foot at home and making cardboard cutouts that you can then slip into shoes in the shop.
- The alternative is to buy your own foot grown gauge. A child's gauge showing UK shoe sizes can be bought mail order £25.95 inc. p&p from Malthouse Hunter Ltd (Tel: 01258 818080).

Shoes

- For babies who are just learning to walk, Daisy Roots 100% soft leather boots (£12, from 0–24 months) are available mail order (Tel: 01604 505611) or through selected shoe shops.
- Bobux shoes (£14.95 a pair) are also available (Tel: 0181 677 9468 for stockists and mail order).

Teeth and Dental Care

As soon as your baby's teeth appear, start cleaning them with an appropriate toothbrush and a minuscule amount of children's toothpaste. This will prevent the build-up of plaque, the main cause of tooth decay.

Checklist
Toothbrushes
- For small babies, look out for 'diamond' headed toothbrushes. Their shape makes it easier for you to clean round the whole mouth.
- Mothers of babies suffering from 'toothbrush fright' reported success in getting junior to open up by using a Fingertip Toothbrush (£1.99, from Tesco Direct).
- It is hard to get toddlers to stand still while brushing their teeth but it is important. (A dentist explained that she had personal experience of toddlers who had fallen over with toothbrushes in their mouths. A fall can cause the toothbrush to become embedded in mouth tissue, sometimes necessitating surgical removal.)
- Musical toothbrushes are often effective in encouraging unwilling toddlers to clean their teeth, though the tunes may have you frothing at the mouth for different reasons.

Toothpaste
- It's the brushing, not the toothpaste, that counts. Too much toothpaste is a bad idea as excessive use of products containing fluoride can affect the appearance of your child's teeth.
- Dentists currently recommend a 'sniff' of a sugar-free toothpaste for milk teeth.

Teething Products

- The Italians use Parmesan rind. Its salty taste and high calcium content make it ideal.
- Cold hard finger foods like frozen bananas may help.
- For really serious teething pain (which includes a temperature and rashes), sugar-free Calpol is usually recommended for babies over three months old.
- See Product Table overleaf for some teething product 'bestsellers', though for some babies nothing seems to work.
- Keep cooling teethers in the fridge but check that you can sterilise any model that you buy for tiny babies and keep these in sterile bags in the fridge. They must be hard and chewable to be of any comfort. Don't 'splash out' on ones filled with water, as small, sharp teeth can burst them.
- For more on rattles/teethers, see p. 195.

Product Table

Toothbrushes

Brand and Price	Comments
My First Colgate Toothbrush (£1.99) ☺	A small toothbrush with a diamond head which is ideal for parents brushing teeth in a small mouth. The best one for a small baby where you are doing the brushing.
Macleans Milk Teeth Toothbrush (£1.79)	A small-headed toothbrush with a good grip, which makes it ideal for either an adult or older baby to use.
Musical Toothbrush (£4.99) ♛	Comes with two heads and batteries included. Suitable from 18 months (from Tesco Direct, Tel: 0345 024024). 'Expensive,' said one parent, 'but a great incentive.'

Toothpastes

Brand and Price	Size and Fluoride Content (parts per million)	Comments
Note: Do not give your child normal toothpaste – it's important to buy a toothpaste formulated for milk teeth.		
Oral B Mint Gel (£1.79)	100ml; 550ppm	Sugar-free, mild mint flavour
My First Colgate (99p)	50ml; 400ppm	Sugar-free, no preservatives, mild mint flavour
Macleans Milk Teeth Training (£1.15)	50ml; 525ppm	Sugar-free, mint flavour, accredited by British Dental Association
Crest Milk Teeth (£1.09)	50ml; 250ppm	Coloured gel, raspberry flavour

Teething Products

Brand	Price and Quantity
Nelson's Teetha Homeopathic Granules	£4.20 for 20 sachets
Boots Sugar-free Teething Gel (birth+)	£1.85 for 15g
Bonjela (three months+)	£2.39 for 15g
Rinstead Teething Gel	£1.85 for 10g

Teething Rings/Keys

Model and Price	Comments
Mam Multi Teether (£3.29)	Has multi-textured patterns on both cooling and hard surfaces.
Mothercare Cooling Teether (£1.99)	A good, hard chunky teether that is easy for small hands to grip.

Teething Rings/Keys (continued)

Model and Price	Comments
Teething Blanket from Blooming Marvellous (£5.99)	A completely new idea for those 'sucky' babies who can't stand life without their security blanket. This is a 100% cotton sheet (32cm×40cm) that has a different-coloured plastic teether at each corner.
Fisher Price Teether 'Key Ring' (£7.95) ☺	A good old-fashioned favourite.

General Baby Goods Suppliers

For specialist suppliers, see relevant chapters.

A number of best buys are stocked by the following multiples. Not all branches carry extensive ranges of baby goods, so it's best to check product availability by phone before you make a special trip.

Multiples

Retailer	Central Office Telephone	Web Site
Argos	0870 600 1010	
Asda	0113 243 5435	www.asda.co.uk
Babies 'R' Us	01628 414141	www.toysrus.co.uk
Boots	0845 070 8090	http://www.boots.co.uk
Children's World	01923 210210	
Ikea	0181 208 5600	www.ikea.com
Index (Littlewoods)	0800 394939	
John Lewis Partnership	0171 828 1000	www.johnlewis.co.uk
Marks & Spencer	0171 935 4422	www.marks-and-spencer.co.uk
Mothercare	01923 210210	
Mothercare World	as above	
Morrisons	01274 494166	
Safeway	0181 848 8744	www.safeway.co.uk
Sainsbury	0171 695 6000	www.j-sainsbury.co.uk
Tesco	0800 505555	www.tesco.co.uk

General Baby Goods Suppliers

Retailer	Central Office Telephone	Web Site
Waitrose	0171 828 1000	as John Lewis

Daisy and Tom may be opening more branches during 1999 but at the moment they can be found in London (Tel: 0171 352 5000) and Manchester (Tel: 0161 835 5000). They do not have a formal mail order service but will gladly post any item requested over the telephone if they have it in stock.

The Baby List Company, The Broomhouse, 50 Sullivan Road, London SW6 (Tel: 0171 371 5145), is an exclusive one-to-one service that will advise and then supply your product requirements.

Mail Order

Retailer	Telephone	Web Site
Boots – Mother and Baby at Home	0845 840 1000	http://www.boots.co.uk.
Blooming Marvellous	0181 391 4822	
Bundles	0151 236 8727	
Cheeky Rascals	01428 682488	
Choice: Mums and Little Ones	0645 100200	
Cotton Moon	0181 305 0012	
Doll's House Emporium	(fax) 01773 513772	
Dragons	0171 589 3795	www.classicengland.co.uk/dragons.html
Early Learning Centre	01793 831300	
English Stamp Company	01929 439117	www.englishstamp.com
Freemans	0800 731 9731	www.freemans.com
Full Moon Futons	0118 926 5648	

Retailer	Telephone	Web Site
Great Little Trading Company	0990 673008	www.gltc.co.uk
Healthy House	01453 752216	
Hill Toy Company	0870 607 1248	hilltoy@prism-dm.co.uk (E-mail only)
JoJo	0171 351 4112	
John Lewis	0171 828 1000	
Kiddycare	01309 674646	
Laura Ashley	01686 622116	
Little Angels	0171 581 1605	
Littlewoods Home Shopping	0345 888 222	
Mark Wilkinson Furniture	01380 850004	
Medela by Mail (Expressions)	01538 386650	
Mini Boden	0181 453 1535	www.boden.co.uk
Mothercare (mail order)	01923 240365	
Mothernature	0161 485 7359	
Nappy Nippas	01736 351263	
NCT Maternity Sales	0141 636 0600	www.nctms.co.uk
Nursery Emporium	01249 811310	www.nursery-emporium.com
Nursery Window	0171 581 3358	
PHP	0870 607 0545	www.medicair.co.uk
Pride and Joy	01721 752686	
Rachel Riley	0171 259 5969	
Red House	01993 779090	www.redhouse.co.uk
Spottiswoode Trading	01903 733123	
Stork Talk	0115 930 6700	
Tesco Baby & Toddler	0345 024024	

General Baby Goods Suppliers

Retailer	Telephone	Web Site
Tridias	0870 240 2104	
Trotters Direct	0990 331188	
Urchin	01672 871515	www.urchin.co.uk
Vertbaudet	0500 332211	www.redoute.co.uk
Video Plus Direct	01733 232800	www.videoplusdirect.com.uk
Waterstone's Books by Post	01225 448595	www.waterstones.co.uk
Wilkinet	01239 841844	

Baby Equipment Hire

The Baby Equipment Hirers' Association (Tel: 01831 310355, or if you have problems getting through: 0113 278 5560) can put you in touch with a local baby equipment hirer.

Regional Retailers

The following shops have been personally recommended by parents for both good service and a good range of baby products. Larger multiples have not been included unless they are either the only shop in a given area or offer consumers a unique service or range of products.

Shop	Address	Telephone
Avon		
Baby Fayre	10–12 Orchard Street, Weston-Super-Mare	01934 418145
The Golden Cot	2 Abbey Street, Bath	01225 263739
Hurwoods	32 Old Market Street, Bristol	01179 279100
Bedfordshire		
Babes Again	5b Riddy Lane, Luton	01582 508946
Baby Bows	64 High Street, Biggleswade	01767 600266
Cyndys	11–12 St Dominics Square, Luton	01582 606449
New Beginnings	28 Brookes Road, Flitwick	01525 719222
Berkshire		
Babywise Buys	Unit 3, 10 Market Street, Bracknell	01344 300390
Bear Necessities	54–70 Moorbridge Road, Maidenhead	01628 778233
W.J. Daniels	Peascod Street, Windsor	01753 862106
Buckinghamshire		
W.A. Childs	202 Desborough Road, High Wycombe	01494 520970
Roses	6 Brunel Centre, Bletchley	01908 630481

Regional Retailers

Shop	Address	Telephone
Scallywags	25 High Street, Stoney Stratford, Milton Keynes	01908 262220
Cambridgeshire		
Baby Plus	15 Chequers Court, Huntingdon	01480 412133
Babycare	34 Burleigh Street, Cambridge	01223 355296
NurseryDays	Burwash Manor Barn, New Road, Barton	01223 264849
Rosie Beginning	Rosie Mat Hospital, Robinson Way, Cambridge	01223 413604
Cheshire		
Baby Face	79A Victoria Street, Crewe	01270 215589
Bambino	3 Hawthorne Lane, Wilmslow	01625 539482
Bambino	6 Kingsway, Altrincham	0161 941 1881
Early Years	596–598 Gorton Road, Reddish, Stockport	0161 231 1900
Hobby Shop	25 Church Street, Runcorn	01928 573614
Nursery World	32 Bramhall Lane, Stockport	0161 480 5688
Toy Town	26 London Road, Stockton Heath, Warrington	01925 261870
Cleveland		
W.H. Watts	114–118 Parliament Road, Middlesbrough	01642 246125
Cornwall		
Adeba Nurseryworld	13 Truro Road, St Austell	01726 73135
Babes and Bikes	8 Polmora Walk, Wadebridge	01208 816282
BabyDays	79 Trelowarren Street, Camborne	01209 718181
Carousel	25–27 Green Lane, Redruth	01209 211298
Keats	7 Princess Street, Bude	01288 355305
Sam's Prams	5 Parade Street, Penzance	01736 364400

Shop	Address	Telephone
County Durham		
Kozi Kids	8 Wesley Street, Consett	01207 506030
Newbies	135 Princess Street, Seaham	0191 581 2396
Cumbria		
Baby World	79 Duke Street, Barrow	01229 822789
Babyworld	113 Strickland Gate, Kendal	01539 740040
Dobie's New Arrivals	104 Senhouse Street, Maryport	01900 813632
Lister's Pram Shop	49 Oxford Street, Workington	01900 601271
Margaret's	59 Highgate, Kendal	01539 722731
Stylewise	70 King Street, Whitehaven	01946 65266
Derbyshire		
Chesterfield Babycare	Brimington Road North, Whittington Moor	01246 454498
Stork Talk (Midlands)	57 South Street, Ilkeston	0115 930 8161
Devon		
W.H. Chope	13–15 High Street, Bideford	01237 472091
Cyril Webber	50 Bear Street, Barnstaple	01271 343277
Exeter Pram and Toys	12 Sidwell Street, Exeter	01392 73119
Kindercare	159 Cowick Street, St Thomas, Exeter	01392 203920
Stork of the Town	42–44 Torwood Street, Torquay	01803 214665
Dorset		
Babygear	33 South Street, Bridport	01308 422522
My Mum's Shop	351 Chickerell Road, Weymouth	01305 779678
Sons and Daughters	382 Ashley Road, Parkstone, Poole	01202 731519
Wiston's	Royal Arcade, Boscombe	01202 393666

REGIONAL RETAILERS

Shop	Address	Telephone
Essex		
Abacus Childrens	75 Cranbrook Road, Ilford	0181 514 4443
Adams Baby Days	97–98 London Road, Benfleet	01268 793674
Babes in the Woods	4 Guildway, South Woodham Ferrers	01245 322266
Baby Basics	279 High Road, Loughton	0181 508 7679
Babycare	9 Rowallen Parade, Green Lane, Dagenham	0181 599 3024
Bear Babies	Wharf Road, Stanford le Hope	01375 361000
Chickadee	87 Ness Road, Shoeburyness	01702 299410
Meryl's Baby 'N' Save	27–30 St Botolph Street, Colchester	01206 766046
Muffets	8 Market Street, Braintree	01376 341519
Pram Craft	4 Station Road, Romford	01708 741991
Sunshine Stores	159 Leigh Road, Leigh-on-Sea	01702 475789
Zebedee	36 Alexandra Street, Southend-on-Sea	01702 351844
Zig Zag	1 Portal Precinct, Sir Isaac Walk, Colchester	01206 766916
Gloucestershire		
Baby Box	4 St Aldate Street, Gloucester	01452 301417
Babyland	52–56 Albion Street, Cheltenham	01242 526862
Hampshire		
Apple of Your Eye	56 The Hundred, Romsey	01794 512737
Baby Care	2 Portland Buildings, Stoke Road, Gosport	01705 583354
Babyneeds Nursery Centre	495 Bitterne Road East, Southampton	01703 434544
Julie's Baby Shop	58 Station Road, New Milton	01425 618199
Kresta	193–199 Kingston Road, Portsmouth	01705 669938

Shop	Address	Telephone
Little Ones	33 Chapel Street, Petersfield	01730 565522
Nurseryland	102 Victoria Road, Aldershot	01252 320487
Oliver's	Oliver's Battery Road South, Winchester	01962 867932
Hertfordshire		
Baby Bits	Jackson Square, Bishop's Stortford	01279 653300
The Hertford Pram Centre	The Malting, Watton Road, Ware	01920 484555
Karen's	1 Bridge Street, Hemel Hempstead	01442 252633
The Nursery Shop	205 Hatfield Road, St Albans	01727 854657
Humberside		
Clothes for Little People	28 Pasture Road, Goole	01405 763071
Hansel and Gretel	57 Toll Gavel, Beverley, Hull	01482 861765
Just Baby	10 Hull Road, Hessie	01482 644117
Kent		
Baby Lady	87 Sea Street, Herne Bay	01227 742586
Babytime	35B Bellegrove Road, Welling	0181 303 2119
Cuddles	20 Bank Street, Herne Bay	01227 387057
Jollytots	116 London Road, Dunton Green, Sevenoaks	01732 742008
Katie's Playpen	1 Pickford Lane, Bexleyheath	0181 303 6313
Kiddiwinks	10 Senacre Square, Wooley Road, Bearsted	01622 681257
Little Rascals	8 London Road, Dover	01504 201299
Little Uns	80 Queen Street, Ramsgate	01843 291069
New Additions	143 High Street, Strood, Rochester	01634 716704
Nippers	Nizels Lane, Hildenborough	01732 832253
Nurseryland	57–59 Upper Dame Road, Margate	01843 292032
Renham's Nursery	11 Cheriton High Street, Cheriton	01303 273832

Regional Retailers

Shop	Address	Telephone
Lancashire		
Nappyline Baby Shop	133 Rochdale Road, Bury	0161 763 4463
Nursery Days	8 Tower Buildings, Leicester Street, Southport	01704 545585
Nurseryworld	157 Victoria Road West, Cleveleys	01253 865562
One Stop Baby Shop	27 Penny Street, Blackburn	01254 674568
Stork Town	5 Market Street, Leigh	01942 677612
Leicestershire		
Baby Barn	Gannow Green Farm, Rubery	01562 710220
Babyquip	107 Uppingham Road, Leicester	0116 274 0573
Prams 'N' Things	108 St Mary's Road, Market Harborough	01858 433775
Lincolnshire		
Moisers	252 Freeman Street, Grimsby	01472 342334
Nurserycare	77 Kruger Street, Spalding	01775 766409
Young World	Compass House, Main Road, Saltfleetby	01507 338266
Youngster's World	1 St George's Road, West Street, Boston	01205 353716
London, East		
All Round Treasures	4 Market Way, Chrisp Street, E14	0171 537 4117
Baby This and That	359 Forest Road, Walthamstow	0181 527 4002
Children's Centre	72–74 Old Church Road, Chingford	0181 529 7465
Gibbons	1–17 Amhurst Road, Hackney	0181 985 3129
Harveys	706 High Road, Leytonstone	0181 539 4538
Jelly Tots	97 Middlesex Street, E1	0171 247 0469
Khalsa	388 Bethnal Green Road, E2	0171 729 3288
Kiddicentre	147 Clapton Common, E5	0181 809 4251

The Best Baby Buys Guide

Shop	Address	Telephone
Salters and Sons	17–19 Barking Road, East Ham	0181 472 2892
London, North		
Infantasia	Units 25–26, Wood Green Shopping City, N22	0181 889 1494
Rubadubdub	198 Stroud Green Road, N4	0171 263 5577
Spoilt Brats	692 High Road, Finchley	0181 445 2505
Totland	4 Bruce Grove, Tottenham	0181 808 3466
London, South		
Bebéworld	191 Balham High Road, Balham	0181 675 8871
Baby World	239 Munster Road, Fulham	0171 386 1904
Lilliput	278 Upper Richmond Road, Putney	0171 780 1682
Lilliput	255 Queenstown Road, SW8	0171 720 5554
Nursery Bargains	19 Westow Street, Upper Norwood	0181 653 9895
G. Swaddlings	21–23 Rushey Green, Catford	0181 897 2992
Tutti Frutti	156–158 Rye Lane, Peckham	0171 732 9933
Wear & Cheer	160 Rye Lane, Peckham	0171 635 9252
London, West		
The Baby List Company (An exclusive one-to-one service that will advise and then supply your product requirements.)	The Broomhouse, 50 Sullivan Road, SW6	0171 371 5145
W.J. Daniel	96–112 Uxbridge Road, Ealing W13	0181 579 1234
Peter Jones	Sloane Square, Chelsea, SW1	0171 730 3434
Manchester		
Colin Bickley	67a Ashton Lane East, Failsworth	0161 681 1944
Cots and Prams	76 Bury Old Road, Whitefield	0161 773 2129
Lesters Discount	4 Bury Old Road, Cheetham Hill Village	0161 720 7227

REGIONAL RETAILERS

Shop	Address	Telephone
Merseyside		
Baby Business	7 The Mount, Heswall, Wirral	0151 342 9970
Formby Prams	37 Three Tuns Lane, Formby	01704 873352
George Henry Lee	20 Basnett Street, Liverpool	0151 709 7070
Scots Nursery World	189 Cantly Road, Walton, Liverpool	0151 523 5991
Middlesex		
Happicraft	48 London Road, Twickenham	0181 892 5262
Kids Klub	38 London Road, Enfield	0181 482 6554
Smarteeland	33 Burnt Oak Broadway, Edgware	0181 200 0370
Waldorfs	Northwick Park Hospital, Watford Road, Harrow	0181 864 7584
Norfolk		
Baby Den	23 St Nicholas Street, Diss	01379 641583
Babyland	1 Wendover Road, New Rackheath, Norwich	01603 722121
Mum's Delight	Mill Barn, Mill Street, Necton, Swaffham	01760 723178
Tots About Town	Magdalen Ind Market, Magdalen Street, Norwich	01603 632613
Northamptonshire		
Kiddiwinks	59–61 Gold Street, Northampton	01604 232241
Nursery Shop	7 Halse Road, Brackley	01280 703838
Northern Ireland		
Diamond Chemist	7 The Diamond, Coleraine, Co. Londonderry	01265 43042
T.G. Hawthorne	7 Thomas Street, Armagh, Co. Armagh	01861 525456
Houston Fashions	Church Street, Ballymena, Co. Antrim	01266 49612
Ivan Jameson	18 High Street, Portadown, Co. Armagh	01762 332244

Shop	Address	Telephone
John McCulloch	18 Bridge Street, Bangor, Co. Down	01247 270443
W.S. Kiddies Corner	The Market House, Unit 1–2 Market Road, Omagh, Co. Tyrone	01662 251108
Linton and Robinson	Abercorn Square, Strabane, Co. Tyrone	01504 382261
MJI Nursery	6 Link Road, Derrychara Industrial Estate, Enniskillen, Co. Fermanagh	01365 323063
The Pram Centre	14 Great James Street, Londonderry	01504 262002
The Pram Shop	38 Castle Street, Belfast	01232 331594
Push Tots	38B Main Street, Castlederg, Co. Tyrone	01662 245178
Sandra's	88 Shore Road, Belfast	01232 770639
Shiels Bros	43 Main Street, Strabane, Co. Tyrone	01504 382681
Toytown	Spencer Road, Londonderry	01504 420011
Toytown	21 Frances Street, Newtownards, Co. Down	01247 819953
Young Additions	77 Main Street, Larne, Co. Antrim	01574 260012
Northumberland		
Baby Needs	30 Bowes Street, Blyth	01670 367632
Nottinghamshire		
Baby and Toddler	34 Station Street, Kirby-in-Ashfield	01623 757810
Oxfordshire		
Junior Citizens	56 Between Towns Road, Cowley	01865 778898
Little Bees	9–11 Mill Street, Wantage	01235 760688
Stork Exchange	6 Greyhound Walk, Thame	01884 218097
Scotland		
Andersons	The Shetland Warehouse, Lerwick	01595 693714
The Baby Castle	Alloway Street, Ayr	01292 262003
Babykins	438 Hillington Road, Glasgow	0141 883 3332

Regional Retailers

Shop	Address	Telephone
Bobtails (Equipment hire.)	11 Lotland, Inverness	01463 242123
Cowan Nursery	Temple Hill, Troon	01292 311211
Duncan MacMillan	80–82 Longrow, Campbeltown	01586 552501
Frasers	99 High Street, Invergordon	01349 852242
Gardiners	48–51 High Street, Brechin	01356 622265
Glasgow Pram Centre	25 McFarlane Street, Glasgow	0141 552 3998
Harris of Saltcoats	106 Dockhead Street, Saltcoats	01294 464330
House & Home	Nursery Corner, Airds Crescent, Oban	01631 565805
Just Kiddin	13 Hanover Street, Stranraer	01776 889445
Just Kidding	10 Canmore Street, Dunfermline	01383 733233
Kenmar	62–64 South Methven Street, Perth	01378 629478
Kidnap	69 Queensberry Street, Dumfries	01387 265019
Little Ones	8 High Street, Galashiels	01898 753308
Little Things	16 Reform Street, Blairgowrie	01250 873335
Mallys	57 Grahams Road, Falkirk	01324 821961
Mathesons	3 Batchen Street, Elgin	01343 542349
The Nappy Pin	62–64 Bonnygate, Cuper	01334 53160
The Nappy Pin	17 Commercial Street, Dundee	01382 221181
Petersons	35–39 High Street, Musselborough	0131 665 2530
Playarama	45 North Bridge Street, Hawick	01450 373352
Raeburn Pram Centre	Stockbridge, Edinburgh	0131 332 8214
Sara's Cottage	Rothesay, Isle of Bute	01700 503280
Shoos Ltd (Excellent range of children's shoes.)	8 Teviot Place, Edinburgh	0131 220 4626
Summers	31 Finlayson Street, Fraserburgh	01346 510228
Wisemans	40 Broad Street, Peterhead	01779 474151

Shop	Address	Telephone
Young Days	23 New Kirkgate, Leith	0131 554 4666
Shropshire		
Newfield Baby Carriages	119a Trench Road, Trench, Telford	01952 70454
Togs For Tots	Royal Shrewsbury Hospital, Maternity Unit	01743 244010
Somerset		
Babes and Tots	6 Bridgwater Road, North Petherton	01278 663271
Banburys	1, 3 and 5 Gold Street, Tiverton	01884 252627
The Children's Cupboard	29 Victoria Street, Burnham on Sea	01278 780300
Staffordshire		
Baby Days	47 Bryan Street, Hanley, Stoke-on-Trent	01782 289109
Suffolk		
Baby Connexions	67 High Street, Haverhill	01440 706292
Bon Bon	19 Hamilton Road, Felixstowe	01394 273663
In Betweens	11 The Traverse, Bury St Edmunds	01284 766383
Surrey		
Baby Room	2 St Martin's Walk, Dorking	01306 887575
Baby's Nest	230 London Road, Croydon	0181 667 9363
The Baby's Room	11 Tunsgate, Guildford	01483 578984
Kid Equip	187 Chipstead Valley Road, Coulsdon	01737 552545
Sussex		
Baby Bargains	2–4 Warren Way, Woodingdean, Brighton	01273 302682
The Baby Shop	19 Springfield Court, Swan Walk, Horsham	01403 218377
Baby Talk	58 North Street, Chichester	01243 779248

Regional Retailers

Shop	Address	Telephone
H.R. Burrell Nursery World	22 Church Road, Burgess Hill	01444 242000
C and N Nursery	31 The Broadway, Crawley	01293 519202
Frills All Round	19–21 Newtown, Uckfield	01825 761625
The Goosebury Bush	2 Barnham Road, Barnham, Bognor Regis	01243 554552
Lullabyes	68–70 Bohemia Road, St Leonard's-on-Sea	01424 423169
Nursery Warehouse	3 Star Road, Old Town, Eastbourne	01323 417775
Over the Rainbow	132 Rectory Road, Worthing	01903 692991
Poppets	50 Blatchington Road, Hove	01273 770449
Sons and Daughters	2 The Parade, East Wittering	01243 670714
Tiny Tribe	25 The Martlets, Burgess Hill	01444 247077
Tyne and Wear		
Bainbridge	Eldon Square, Newcastle	0191 232 5000
Fenwick Ltd	Northumberland Street, Newcastle	0191 232 5100
Joanna Toys	32 Front Street, Monkseaton	0191 252 9984
Mothercare World	Team Valley Trading Estate, Gateshead	0191 491 0080
Nursery Thyme	2 Bridge Street, Sunderland	0191 567 0534
Wales		
Beehive Babyworld	74 Chester Road East, Shotton	01244 811080
Beryl Jones	5 Commercial Street, Risca	01633 612749
Candid Cards	31 Church Street, Flint	01352 732532
Cardiff Buggy Clinic (Buggies fixed. Ring before you go to see if it can be done while you wait.)	226 Cowbridge Road West, Cardiff	01222 575969

Shop	Address	Telephone
W.J. Daniel	2–12 City Road, Cardiff	01222 452894
Dorina	Dimond Street, Pembroke Dock	01646 683174
Eddershaws	Phoenix Way, Enterprise Park, Swansea	01792 774400
Hurwoods Nursery World	36 Sovereign Arcade, Kingsway Centre, Newport	01633 246448
R.A. Jones	37 High Street, Caernarfon	01286 673121
J.T. Morgan	12–24 Belle Vue Way, Swansea	01792 655231
The Nursery Shop	Main Road, Llawtwir Fardre, Pontypridd	01443 204192
The Pram Shop	12 New Street, Neath	01639 643108
Warwickshire		
Kidding Around	17 St John's, Warwick	01926 492888
West Midlands		
Jolly Tots	41 Stoney Lane, Yardley, Birmingham	0121 789 6646
Just Kidding	Stone Yard, Digbeth	0121 622 3100
Kiddisave	Seymour House, Green Lane, Walsall	01922 626466
Wiltshire		
Nursery Rhymes	4 Cross Keys Chequer, Salisbury	01722 412872
Nursery Tymes	Couch Lane, Devizes	01380 721747
Worcestershire		
Pauline's	22 West Street, Leominster	01568 613193
Yorkshire		
Baby Care	75 Town Street, Armley	01232 319165
Babycare	1 Junction Terrace, Bolton Road, Bradford	01274 640364
Babycentre	MAM House, Roseville Road, Leeds	0113 245 5680
Baby Days	235 Sprotsborough Road, Doncaster	01302 391420

Regional Retailers

Shop	Address	Telephone
Babyland (Service engineer on site to repair brand name buggies.)	13 Petersgate, Bradford	01274 394387
H. Brown	15 Roper Gate, Pontefract	01977 703726
Kaleidoscope	1 Somerset Terrace, Scarborough	01723 351305
Little Joe's	25 Northway, Scarborough	01723 351702
Paul Stride	7 Acomb Court, Front Street, Acomb, York	01904 798536
Sitsafe Babycentre	Bradford Road, Stockbridge, Keighley	01535 681021
Stead's of York	74 Goodram Gate, York	01904 624335
The Stork	10 Market Road, Doncaster	01302 364462
Toyland Too	16 Newmarket, Otley	01942 467417

Index

activity centres 194, 197
all-terrain buggies 117, 135-6
allergies 77
American products 8
antiseptic sprays 87
armbands 146

baby carriers 11, 153-7
  back carriers 153, 155, 156-7
  front carriers 153, 154, 155
  hip, resting on 156
baby clothes 19-28
  bodysuits 19, 22, 25, 26
  bootees and shoes 22, 242-3
  cardigans/sweatshirts 22, 23, 27, 28
  checklist 20-3
  christening wear 23
  for crawlers and toddlers 27-8
  dungarees 26
  easy-care garments 20-1
  fabrics 21
  gowns 21-2
  hand-made woollens 23
  hangers 24
  jogpants and trousers 26, 27, 28
  mittens 22, 23
  for newborns 25-6
  for premature babies 26-7
  product tables 25-8
  pyjamas and nighties 23
  shopping list 19-20
  size guide 23-4
  snowsuits 22-3
  socks 22, 25
  stretchsuits/sleepsuits/babygrows 21, 25, 26, 27
  sun hats 141, 143
  for sunny holidays 142
  swimwear 142, 144, 145
  T-shirts 26, 142, 144
  trainer pants 225
  underwear 28
  vests 22, 25, 26, 27
Baby Equipment Hirers Association 140
'Baby Gift List' services 6
baby lotion 35
baby oil 35
Baby Products Association (BPA) 4, 12
baby rice 207
baby walkers 152
babygrows *see* stretchsuits
balcony guards 234
balloons 189
bandages 87
bath mats, non-slip 29, 30, 31
bath products 30, 34-5
  baby lotion 35
  bath temperature thermometers 35, 234
  bath toys 35, 196
  shampoo 35
  soap and bubble bath 34
  sponges 34

INDEX

talcum powder 35
towels 30, 34
bath rings 29, 31
bath supports 29, 30-1, 32
bathroom safety 232, 234
baths 29-35
- bath seats 33
- bath stand 31
- in changing units 31, 65, 66-7
- check list 30-1
- for new babies 32-3
- for older babies 33
- portable baths 33
- product table 32-3
- shopping list 30
- that fit on top of your own 30, 32
- top and tail bowl 29
- traditional baths 30, 32
- tummy tubs 30, 33

bedding 79-82
- blankets 79, 81, 82
- cot bumper 80
- mattress protectors 76, 80, 82
- sheets 80, 81, 82
- sleeping bags 79
- things *not* to buy 80
- wedges 80

bibs 215-16
blankets 79, 81, 82
bodysuits 19, 22, 25, 26
boiler vents 234
books 162-68, 224
- age and development 162
- book list 164-7
- mail order 167
- on tape 168

bootees 22
bottle carriers 48
bottle feeding 15, 36-42
- Avent system 38, 42
- bottle capacity 37
- disposable bottle systems 37-8, 42
- formula 36-7
- on holiday 140
- on the move 36, 50
- powder dispensers 50
- product table 41-3
- self-sealing caps 41, 43
- shaped bottles 37
- shopping list 36
- standard bottles 37, 40-1
- wide-neck bottles 37, 41-2
- *see also* sterilisers; teats

bottle-feeding accessories 48-50
- bottle carriers 48
- bottle and teat brushes 48
- bottle warmers 49, 50

bouncers 149-50
- doorframe model 12, 149, 151
- free standing 149-51

bowls 210-11, 212-13
- stay-warm bowls 211
breast packs 61
breast pads 59, 60-1
breast pumps 62-4
- battery/mains-powered 63, 64
- electric 62, 63, 64
- manual 62, 63-4

breast shells 59-60, 61
breastfeeding accessories 59-61
- breast packs 61
- breast pads 59, 60-1
- breast shells 59-60, 61
- nipple creams 60
- nipple shields 60

breastfeeding bras 53-8
- drop-cup 54, 56-7
- front-opening 55, 57
- size 55-6
- sleep bras 55, 58

zip-cup 55, 57-8
breastfeeding counsellors 53
breastfeeding on holiday 137
British Standards Institute (BSI) 12
bubble bath 34
buggies *see* pushchairs and buggies
building bricks 198

calamine lotion 87
car activity centres/play trays 112, 113
car seat accessories 111-13
car seats 11, 103-10
    backward facing 104-5, 106
    booster seats 107-08, 110
    fitting 104
    forward facing 104, 107-8, 108, 109-10
    infant carriers 104, 106, 108-9
    integral seats 104
    product tables 108-10
    seat sizes and styles 103-5, 106-8
    three-way seats 106-7
    twins and triplets 14
    two-way seats 104, 105, 106
car sleep cushions 113
car sunshades 112
cardigans 22, 23
carrycots *see* pushchairs and buggies
catalogue stores 6
Centre for Accessible Environments (CAE) 16
chain stores 6
chairs 158-61
    bouncy chairs 13, 158-60
    headhuggers 159, 160
    highchairs 217-23
    swinging chairs 12, 160-1
changing accessories 101-2
changing bags 15, 48, 172-5
changing mats 65, 66, 68, 173
changing units 65-8
    integral bath 31, 65, 66-7
christening wear 23
cleaning fluids 232
competitions and special offers 8
computers *see* multimedia
consumer testing 4
cooker guard 231, 236
cot bumpers 80
cot death (Sudden Infant Death Syndrome) 75, 79, 80, 93
cots and cot beds 13, 14, 69-74, 84
    bedside cots 84
    carrycots 126, 127, 129, 199
    comparisons 69-70
    cot activity centres 194
    cribs and cradles 70, 71, 73
    drop-sides 70, 72, 73
    product table 71-3
    safety 71, 74
    second-hand 74
    skycots 139
    teething rails 70, 72, 73
    travel cots 199-201
    see also mattresses
cotton buds 35
cotton wool pads 34
crayons 198
cribs and cradles 70-1, 73
cups 211, 213-14
curtains and blinds 183, 186-7
cycling with a baby 176-80

INDEX

child seats 176, 177-78, 179, 180
  cycle helmets 176, 177, 179
  sidecars 178
  trailers 178, 179

decongestants 87
dimmer switches 181, 183
Disabled Living Foundation 15, 16
doll's house items 185
domestic alterations 16
door slam stoppers 14, 235
double buggies 132-4
  alternatives to 132
  side-by-sides 132, 134
  tandems 133, 134
dummies *see* soothers
dungarees 26

edge cushions 230, 235
electrical safety 229, 231, 232, 235
European baby product standards 12

fences and garden gates 233
fire retardants 77
fire safety 181, 229, 235
fireguards 181, 229, 235
first aid kits 86, 138, 236
float suits 145-6
food 205-9
  baby rice 207
  commercial baby foods 205, 206-8
  commercial ingredients 206-7
  freezing 206, 208
  fruit drinks 209
  home-cooked 205, 206, 208
  organic baby foods 206
  storage containers 208-9
  weaning 205-6, 207
  whole-milk products 206
  see also bottle feeding
food warmers 50
foreign goods 9
formula 37-8
Foundation for the Study of Infant Deaths (FSID) 75, 79, 80
fruit drinks 209
furniture corners 230, 235
furniture, nursery 181, 183, 185

garden safety 233-4
garden toys 198, 233
gates and barriers 237-41
  garden 233
  stair gates 239-41
glass 230, 236
  safety glass 230
gowns 21-2
grants 15
Great Little Trading Company 8
'Great Value Buy' 5

hangers 24
harnesses 9, 236
  see also individual products
heating 181, 184
  fan heaters 181, 184
  thermostatic controls 181, 184
  wall-mounted radiators 184
highchairs 13, 217-23
  booster seats 220, 222
  checklist 20-3
  convertible/cube 219
  folding 219, 221, 222
  folding high/low chairs 219, 221

harness 218, 223
portable/table-top 219, 222
problems 217-18
product table 221-3
rigid/traditional 219, 221-3
safety 220
screw-on models 220, 222
seat 218
second-hand 223
storage and portability 218
toys 223
travel highchairs 14
tray 218
hire services 140, 251
holidays 137-46
family-friendly tour operators 139-40
float suits 145-6
floats and armbands 146
hiring equipment 140
holiday packs 146
insect repellant 142
packing list 137-9
sun protection 141-2, 143, 144
swimwear 142, 144, 145-6
tents and cabanas 141, 143
travel necessities 139
homeopathic remedies 88
Hospital Pack 26

in-car entertainment and storage 112
in-car food and drink storage 112
insect repellant 142
instruction leaflets 10
Internet: shopping online 8

jogpants 26

kitchen safety 231-2, 235-6
kitemark 192

lighting
dimmer switches 181, 183
nightlights 90, 181, 184, 229
sockets 184
lion mark 192
locks 10
doors/cabinets 229, 231, 235
kitchen equipment 235-6
toilet 232, 234
windows 230, 236
'Luxury Buy' 5

mail order shopping 7-8
suppliers 249-51
matching and sorting games 198
maternity wear 8
mattress protectors 75, 80, 82
mattresses 11, 75-8, 200
allergies 77
cleaning 76, 77
fire retardants 77
fit 75
foam/ventilated foam 75, 76
natural fibres 76-7
prams 123
product table 77-8
spring interior 76
thickness 75
medicine cabinet 87-8
medicine droppers 87
micropore tape 87
mitten clips 22
mittens 22, 23
mobiles 189, 193
monitors 5, 89-93

INDEX

integral night light 90, 92, 184
low-volume feature 91, 92
plug-in 89, 91-2
portable 90, 92
rechargeable 90, 92-3
two channels 90-1, 92
video 90, 93
visual indicator 91, 92
Moses baskets 15, 83-5
multimedia 171
musical toys 194, 197
muslin squares 101

nail cutters/scissors 87
nappies 94-100
   biodegradable liners 98
   bulk buying 95, 96
   disposable 15, 95, 96-7
   disposal bags 96
   ecological factors 94
   home delivery 7, 95, 96-7
   nappy bin 96
   nappy services 94, 99-100
   night time 95
   reusable 94, 98-100
   shaped 98-99
   swim nappies 145
   terry 98
   see also changing accessories
nappy rash cream 87, 101
National Nursery Education Board (NNEB) 4
nighties 23
nightlights 90, 181, 184, 229
Nippers 6-7, 9
nipple creams 60
nipple shields 60
nursery 181-8
   furniture 181, 183, 185
   heating 184
   lighting 181, 182, 183-4
   nursery toys 185
   product tables 185-8
   safety 182
   shopping list 181
   storage 181, 183
   wall decorations 187-8
   wallpapers and soft furnishings 183, 186-7
   see also cots and cot beds; monitors
nursery characters, self-adhesive 187

out of town retailers 6
oven guard 231

paints and varnishes 10, 74
   paint stripping 182
Pampers Parenting Institute 8
paracetamol, infant 87
pet faeces 233
pillows 80
plasters 87
play gyms 196
play mats 194-5
ponds and pools 233
potties 13, 224-5, 226-7
   musical/novelty potties 225, 226
   travel potties 227
prams 123-4
   manufacturers 121-2, 124
   mattresses 123
pregnancy and baby magazines 8
premature baby clothes 26-7
print blocks 188
pull-along toys 198
pushchairs and buggies 114-36
   accessories 115, 120-1
   after-sales care 118
   all-terrain buggies 115, 135-6

brakes 117
buggies/strollers 114, 115, 117, 127, 130-1, 138
buying overseas 117
carrycots 126, 127, 129, 199
changing bags 115
checklists 116-20, 126-7
combination (three-in-one) 114, 126, 128-9
convertibles (two-in-one) 114, 126, 127-9
cost and quality 116-7
discounts and bargains 117-8
double buggies 132-4
fabrics 118
folding mechanisms 116, 118-9
foot muff/cosytoes 120
handles 119, 128
harness 120
hiring 115
manufacturers 121-2
product tables 127-31
safety 117
seat options 119, 126, 128, 129, 130
second-hand 120
shopping tray 116, 119
strollers 131
sun canopy 120, 121, 128, 129, 142
travel systems 114, 115, 126-7, 129-30
for twins and triplets 13-14, 115-6
umbrella-fold stroller 115, 117, 127, 130-1, 138
waterproof cover 121, 130
weight and size 118
wheels and suspension 119

see also prams
pushing/riding toys 197-8
puzzles 197
pyjamas 23

rail nets 231, 234
rattlers and teethers 195
rear-seat/child view mirrors 111-12
rocking horses 185
rugs 230

safety 4
  BS/CE mark 12
  danger checklist 229-34
  Save a Baby's Life (training sessions) 228
  see also individual products
safety gadgets 14, 228-36
  baby-proofing service 228
  balcony guards 234
  bath thermometers 35, 234
  cooker guard 231, 236
  edge cushions 230, 235
  harnesses 9, 236
  locks *see* locks
  oven guard 236
  product table 234-6
  rail nets 231, 234
  smoke alarms 182, 236
  socket plugs and covers 14, 182, 229, 235
  tap covers 35, 232, 234
  video guards 236
second-hand equipment 8-12
  checking 8-11
  'nearly new' shops 9
  sample prices 12
  sources 9
  unsuitable products 11
  see also individual products

INDEX

shampoo 35
shawls 23, 80
sheets 80, 81, 82
   mattress protectors 75, 80, 82
   pram sheets 123
shoes 22, 242-3
shopping incentives/bargain buys 6
sidecars, cycle 178
skin cream 87
sleeping bags 79
sleepsuits *see* stretchsuits
smoke alarms 182, 236
snowsuits 22-3
soap 34
Social Services 15
socket plugs and covers 14, 182, 229, 235
socks 22, 25
soft toys 195-6
soothers/dummies 51-2
special needs babies 15-16
specialist baby shops 6-7
sponges 34
spoons 210, 212
stair gates 239-41
stairs 231, 235
standards for baby products 12
stationary entertainers 152
stencils 188
sterile dressings 87
sterilisers 15, 43-7
   bottle compatibility 43
   capacity and size 43-4
   checklist 43-5
   chemical sterilisers 44, 45-6
   microwave sterilisers 44, 45, 47
   product table 45-7
   steam sterilisers 44, 46
   tongs 45, 46
story tapes 168
stretchsuits/sleepsuits/babygrows 19, 21, 25, 26, 27
strollers *see* pushchairs and buggies
sun canopy 120, 121, 128, 129, 142
sun hats 141, 143
sun protection 141-4
sunscreen 142, 144
sunshades (cars) 112
suppliers 6-8
   mail order 7-8, 249-51
   multiples 6, 248-9
   regional retailers 252-65
sweatshirts 22, 27, 28
swimseats 146
swimwear 142, 143, 145-6

T-shirts 26, 142, 144
tables 230
talcum powder 35
tap covers 35, 232, 234
teats 38-42
   anti-colic valves 39, 41, 42
   brushes 48
   flow 39
   latex teats 39, 40, 41
   materials 39
   orthodontic teats 39, 51
   ribbed teats 39
   silicone teats 15, 37, 38, 39, 40, 41, 42
   wide-neck teats 39
   see also soothers
Teddies Nurseries 4
teeth and dental care 244-7
   teething products 245, 246
   teething rings/keys 195, 246-7
   toothbrushes 30, 245, 246
   toothpaste 30, 244, 246
teething blanket 247

teething gel 87
teething products 246, 247
teething rings/keys 195, 246-7
tents and cabanas 141, 143, 198
thermometers
  baby's thermometer 88
  bath thermometer 35, 234
  room thermometer 80-1, 181
toilet locks 232, 234
toilet training aids 224-7
  foldaway loo seat 225, 227
  potties 224-5, 226-7
  toilet seat adaptors 225
  trainer pants 225
toiletries *see* bath products
toothbrushes 30, 245, 246
toothpaste 30, 244, 246
towels 30, 34
toxic plants 234
toy libraries 189
toys 189-98
  age and development 191-2
  age warning symbol 193
  bath toys 35, 196
  for car travel 112, 113
  garden toys 233
  highchair toys 223
  nursery toys 185
  product tables 193-5
  safety 190
  shopping list 189-90
  standards 192-3
  see also individual toys
trailers, cycle 178, 179

trainer pants 225
travel cots 12, 199-201
  folding cots 199, 201
  packaway cots 199, 200-1
  second-hand 200
travel systems *see* pushchairs and buggies
trousers 27, 28
tummy tubs 30, 33
Twins and Multiple Births Association (TAMBA) 13
twins and triplets 12-15, 21
  car seats 14
  equipment 13-15
  pushchairs and buggies 13-14, 115-6, 132-4

underwear 28

'Very Popular Buy' 5
vests 22, 25, 26, 27
video guards 236
videos 169-70

wall hangings 188
wallpapers and soft furnishings 181, 186-7
washing powders and conditioners 21
weaning 205-6, 207
  see also bowls; cups; spoons
wedges 80
window bars 230
window locks 230, 236
wipes 101-2
woollens, hand-made 23

Young Book Trust 163

Readers' Report Form

If you have best buys, hints, tips or news of disastrous purchases you want to pass on to other parents, please let us know either by E-mailing us on book4baby@aol.com or posting this form, post free, to: Juliet Leigh, Dennis Reed Research, FREEPOST, 172 Greenford Road, Harrow, Middlesex HA1 3BR.

Your name ....

Address ....

....

....

Telephone ....

Product ....

Where you bought it ....

Comments ....

....

....

....

....

....